Hormone

A Matter of Life and Health

BALANCE

A Comprehensive
Guide to Natural
Hormone Balance
for Women
and Health
Care Professionals

Kristine B. Klitzke, R.N., B.S.N

D1280332

Hormone Balance:

A Matter of Life and Health

A Comprehensive Guide to Natural Hormone Balance for Women and Health Care Professionals.

Version 2

Kristine B. Klitzke, R.N., B.S.N

Published by
Sound Concepts, Inc.
15 East 400 South
Orem, Utah 84058
(801)-225-9520 / (800)-544-7044

Table of Contents

Section One
A Message to the Medical Community

Section Two
Hormones and Hormone Imbalance: An Overview

Section Three
The Hormone Factor:
<u>Conditions and Symptoms of Estrogen Dominance</u>

Section Four
A Cancer Growing Among Us

Section Five
A Message About Menopause

Section Six
Final Thoughts

Section Seven
Appendices

Acknowledgments

Special thanks to Donna Johnson for inspiring me to write this book. Your positive spirit and guidance have been especially encouraging to me along the entire journey.

Sincere thanks to my brother-in-law, Doug Klitzke for his valuable input. Doug generously contributed an enormous amount of his time and expertise in painstakingly critiquing my final drafts. Doug's intelligence and insight provided me with numerous helpful suggestions in the areas of punctuation, sentence structure, and word choice. I am extremely grateful for Doug's ability to zero in on ways to improve my book's readability and professionalism.

Genuine thanks and appreciation to Dr. Robert Gottesman, M.D. Although Dr. Gottesman and I had never formally met, he selflessly agreed to read my manuscript and offer his professional advice. Dr. Gottesman generously gave of his time and shared his expertise to improve the readability of my book on a medical level. Dr. Gottesman's contributions from a medical standpoint were instrumental in strengthening the credibility and accuracy of my work.

My sincere appreciation also goes out to the loving members of my family and wonderful friends who have given me words of encouragement, provided me with help in caring for Leah and Kalen, and kept me focused on my priorities along the way. There are too many of you to mention – you know who you are. I cherish you in my life.

To my husband, Brad, and daughters, Leah and Kalen, I express my deep love and thankfulness. Your constant supply of smiles and hugs in the midst of my moments of frustration during the writing of this book brought me much joy. Most of all, I am grateful for your patience and unconditional love. You are such blessings to me.

Finally, with my whole heart, I give thanks to my Heavenly Father. Through His grace, He has blessed me with the passion, vision, and strength to see this "labor of love" to completion while keeping me in His perfect peace.

Dedication

Dedicated to all the women who have shared with me how the important truths regarding hormone balance have changed their lives and health. It is because of your experiences that I have persevered in completing this book. I know that just as these truths have offered each of you hope and health, they will do so for countless others as well.

Foreword

You are about to discover that the author of this book is no ordinary medical professional. Kristine Klitzke is one of those rare birds that are able to leave the flock and fly alone. Kris' intense passion and ability to effectively communicate the truth about hormones and how hormone balance affects our lives and health could help thousands of individuals achieve optimal wellness and perhaps even save lives. The reason behind Kris' desire for writing this book is simply that she wants to share what she has learned in order that others may benefit. Kris is gifted with the ability to share her knowledge so that other health care professionals as well as laypersons will be able to understand and utilize the concepts she describes.

I have personally observed Kris' transformation as she discovered the magnitude that hormone imbalance issues are involved in numerous health symptoms and conditions as well as the truth found in natural progesterone therapy. Kris' priority has always been to deliver only the most current, accurate information. Doing so, involved enormous amounts of research. Despite maintaining a busy household with two preschool aged daughters, Kris would stay up late into the night, pouring hundreds of hours into research and study, compiling the latest medical information from recognized medical journals and experts in the field.

Eventually, Kris began sharing her knowledge by organizing "Health Awareness Seminars" at the local hospital she has been employed with since receiving her Bachelor of Science Degree in Nursing in 1990. With a fervent passion for the topic at hand, Kris delivered educational messages to those who attended these lectures. In addition to lecturing, Kris also provided informational handouts on a variety of related topics. Her handouts became extremely popular and it was from these handouts that I realized Kris "had a book inside of her."

The morning after one of Kris' hospital lectures I called her to suggest that she organize her information and publish a book. Kris took my suggestion to heart and immediately embarked on her book, mostly in the wee hours of the night as her young family slept. Tired as she was, Kris' thoughts kept flowing and her fingers kept typing. Inspired by the latest news stories and relevant research pertinent to her topic, as well as a dose of divine intervention, Kris has been able to complete this valuable work.

In the movie, "Pay it Forward," we saw how helping one person and asking them to "pay it forward," was able to influence the world on a magnificent level. After reading *"Hormone Balance: A Matter of Life and Health,"* I encourage you to pass the information on. By passing it on, Kris' labor will be rewarded. Share it with those you care about, including your health care provider. I have heard it said that, "knowledge is not power, but rather information to make wise choices." Empower yourself with the truth, enabling you to make informative health care decisions. Then, "pay it forward!"

Donna Johnson

Introduction

Dear Reader,

My interest in women's health issues, as they relate to hormone balance, began early in the year 2000 when I was invited by a neighbor to attend a wellness class. It was at this class that I was first introduced to the numerous and significant ways hormone balance can affect our lives and health.

Admittedly, I was a bit skeptical upon hearing a description of the numerous predominant health concerns that can result from a type of hormone imbalance known as *estrogen dominance*, the many risks involved with prescribed synthetic hormone use, and the benefits possible by restoring balance to estrogen and progesterone levels. I was never educated on these concepts in nursing school or through any continuing education curriculum during my nursing career. Nonetheless, I was left intrigued by the possibility that while most health concerns develop as a result of multiple factors, the "hormonal factor" was an important piece of the puzzle frequently overlooked.

As a registered nurse since 1990, I have witnessed an overwhelming number of individuals (usually females) experience a number of disturbing health concerns which have become quite commonplace. These include pelvic disorders which often result in a hysterectomy (such as abnormal bleeding, endometriosis, fibroids, and ovarian cysts), thyroid disorders, and cancer (especially of the breast, cervix, ovaries, and prostate). I have also been perplexed at the ever-increasing number of individuals (again, usually *females*) who are diagnosed with conditions like fibrocystic breasts, migraine headaches, fibromyalgia, chronic fatigue syndrome, autoimmune diseases, unexplained weight gain, and others.

Finally, it's been of concern to me that women taking prescribed synthetic hormones, either in the form of chemical contraceptives (such as the birth control pill) or hormone replacement therapy, frequently experience a variety of side effects – some quite serious. For years I questioned to myself why these drugs are so routinely prescribed, while at the same time, are immediately discontinued with a suspected or confirmed diagnosis of cancer. Regrettably, I never took the time to consider the reasons behind these disturbing observations until recently.

With books in hand from the public library as well as medical journals from the hospital library, little did I realize that I was about to embark upon what would become my new "platform." Before long, my eyes were opened to a logical explanation of the factors contributing to the widespread presence of estrogen dominance, a form of hormone imbalance whereby estrogen is in excess (the "dominant" hormone) relative to progesterone levels. I also discovered the physiological basis behind how estrogen dominance can contribute to the development of numerous unfavorable symptoms and conditions in otherwise healthy individuals. In addition, I began researching the rationale behind the benefits of restoring hormone balance naturally.

In the process, I was overwhelmed by the amount of research available regarding the risks associated with prescribed synthetic hormone use in the forms of chemical contraceptives and hormone replacement drugs. Of paramount importance to me, was the fact that everything I was learning made *sound, physiological sense*. It was at this juncture that I acquired a whole new respect for and understanding of just how intricately hormones, both endogenous (manufactured within the body) and exogenous (introduced from outside the body), can affect our lives and health.

For medical personnel in particular, this information could prove to be extremely valuable in diagnosing, treating, and most importantly, for preventing a variety of common, and oftentimes serious, health concerns. Realizing how uninformed and even misinformed I, a health care professional, had been regarding the numerous and significant ways hormones affect us, it was impossible for me to keep the information to myself. The more I learned, the more I desired for others to know as well. It has been my pleasure to communicate this message by giving public lectures since the summer of 2000. On a similar note, I'm thrilled to be able to share what I have learned about these topics via the power of the written word.

It is my hope that *"Hormone Balance: A Matter of Life and Health"* will offer a clear and sound explanation of the conditions often related to the hormone imbalance situation known as estrogen dominance, the potential risks involved with the use of prescribed synthetic hormones (chemical contraceptives and hormone replacement therapy), and the rationale supporting how natural progesterone therapy is capable of preventing and correcting conditions that can occur throughout a woman's lifetime from an environment of estrogen dominance by restoring hormone balance. Other themes woven throughout the text focus on the preventative aspects of medicine and the importance of diagnosing and correcting the underlying causes of health conditions versus the practice of eliminating symptoms only (symptom-based treatment).

While this publication is the product of my sincere desire to convey the critical truths regarding hormones and hormone balance to people in *all* walks of life, I have included an enormous amount of data based on the latest research and clinical findings that will be of particular interest to health care professionals.

My thanks and appreciation go out to everyone who takes a moment to give these sound and profound concepts a second thought!

With warm regards,

Kristine Klitzke RN, BSN

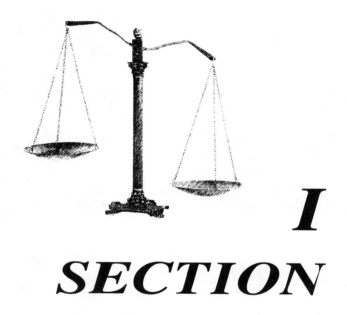

I
SECTION

A Message to the
Medical Community

ONE   **1**

Dear Doctor...

Interestingly, among the 29 chapters I have written for this book, this is the chapter I found most difficult to write! It has been a struggle for me to adequately communicate the fact that while I respect and value a variety of aspects of the medical profession, at the same time I am convinced that there are some areas of medicine that need to be approached differently.

The message I desire to convey to the medical community involves several important themes regarding the impact of hormones and hormone balance on the lives and health of women. My hope is that by understanding the concepts I describe, the medical community will approach a number of predominant female health concerns with a different perspective – one by which the likelihood of hormones *and* hormone imbalance are considered as possibly playing major roles. With this approach, steps would be taken to prevent or treat health concerns by identifying and eliminating known sources of potentially harmful hormonal agents (estrogens, estrogenic compounds, and progestins). At the same time, in cases of suspected or confirmed estrogen dominance, natural progesterone therapy would be considered as a way to counteract estrogen's effects and restore the body's progesterone levels, ultimately promoting hormone balance.

The "Hormone Connection"

Like many health care professionals, I have been perplexed by the ever-increasing incidences of women presenting with pelvic disorders (irregular bleeding, endometriosis, ovarian cysts, cervical dysplasia, and uterine fibroids), thyroid conditions (often resulting in weight gain, depression, loss of libido, and fatigue), and cancer of the breast, ovaries, and cervix. Even more perplexing has been the fact that it is not the traditionally depicted "older woman" presenting with these conditions on a more frequent basis but *younger* women between the ages of 30 and 50. Even those in their teens and twenties are increasingly affected as well. In addition, it has been disconcerting to encounter such a high number of individuals plagued by challenging conditions such as frequent headaches, fibromyalgia, chronic fatigue syndrome, and autoimmune diseases – primarily women.

Although physicians and other health care professionals acknowledge these same observations in their own practices, the possibility of hormones playing a pivotal role in the underlying etiologies may be overlooked. Yet, a common thread in explaining the origins of many of these health concerns can be traced back to "hormone imbalance"- specifically that of *estrogen dominance*, a condition in the body whereby estrogen levels are in excess relative to progesterone. In addition, it is more than a coincidence that the health histories of a significant percentage women affected by these health concerns often reflect a current or past use of some form of prescribed synthetic hormone.

While most health symptoms and conditions are multi-factorial in origin, the roles of hormones and hormone imbalance are clearly worth considering in a variety of symptoms and conditions suffered by women for years. Also, the logic of restoring hormone balance in an environment of estrogen dominance by eliminating known sources of exogenous estrogen and raising progesterone levels with *natural* progesterone merits attention. In the same way, the benefits of using natural progesterone as a safe and effective alternative to traditionally prescribed hormone replacement for managing menopausal symptoms warrant recognition.

A Female Patient's Perspective

While I have no doubt that physicians always have their patients' best interests in mind, as a result of my interactions with women the past several years of lecturing on women's health issues, I have identified some specific areas of concern regarding health care that women consistently bring to my attention.

Like other health care professionals, I have witnessed many of the risk factors surrounding the use of prescribed synthetic hormones come to fruition time and time again in patients I encounter in the preoperative setting. Yet, these drugs continue to be routinely prescribed until the first sign of danger (often a suspected or confirmed malignancy), upon which it is prudent practice to immediately discontinue them. The familiar scenario involves a woman taking the birth control pill or HRT who discovers a lump in her breast.

Because the estrogens and progestins commonly found in these medications are known carcinogens (placed on the Federal List of Carcinogenic Substances in 1988 and 2000 respectively), she is immediately advised to refrain from taking further doses pending subsequent test results. This practice has been a source of confusion as well as concern for many of the women who have experienced it first-hand. Because of what is now known about traditionally prescribed synthetic hormones, women today are interested in more natural therapies when seeking to prevent or treat their health problems.

Women also express concern with "symptom-based treatment," the practice of prescribing synthetic hormones or other drugs specifically to eliminate their symptoms in lieu of diagnosing and correcting underlying conditions – many of which are associated with hormone imbalance. For example, when a woman experiences severe menstrual cramping or heavy menstrual bleeding, it has become common practice to prescribe the birth control pill in order to eliminate her symptoms by eliminating her natural menstrual cycle all together. However, most women are no longer interested in the "quick-fix" but rather in having the underlying causes of their health concerns identified and corrected – a practice by which conservative yet complete healing can often take place with the restoration of hormone balance and positive lifestyle changes.

A final point I wish to highlight on behalf of female patients is that although I encourage women to discuss the roles hormones and hormone balance can play in their health with their health care providers, it never ceases to amaze me that a number of women, fearing a negative reception, are reluctant to even bring the subject up with them. Unfortunately for some women, these fears are validated as they are met with hostility at the mere mention of it.

While responses vary, many women encounter a lack of support from physicians when discussing the concept of hormone imbalance playing an intricate roll in their health concerns. In addition, the prospect of using natural progesterone to restore hormone balance is met with skepticism despite medical data supporting its safety and efficacy. Even physicians, like Jacques Roussouw, who have become skeptical of prescription synthetic hormones, face hostility among colleagues. Roussouw, acting director of the huge Women's Health Initiative, which has discovered significant risks with conventional hormone replacement therapy, explains, "I talk to gynecologists, trying to lay out the pros and cons (of HRT), and I often get quite a hostile reception for being skeptical." Personally, I can relate to the fact that no matter what the subject is, if it is something I have not thoroughly researched for myself, I tend to have more of a negative opinion of it.

With busy practices, physicians have shared what a challenge it can be to routinely take in the latest books, articles, and research published in recognized medical journals on these and related topics. Instead, the brochures and informational bits distributed by drug companies that flood a physician's mail daily tend to be read on a regular basis. While often leading to a bias or "slant" on the information provided to physicians, this is the information that ultimately influences many decisions surrounding patient health care concerns.

An Integrative Approach

Years ago, the "medical approach" to health and well-being was not the predominant health care system it is today, but rather an equal choice among many including chiropractic, homeopathy, and others. Each was recognized and considered for its individual value in health maintenance, prevention, and potential cures. However, since the advent of pharmaceuticals, we seemed to have lost sight of the significance those other aspects of care can have. We need to recognize once again how both conventional and complementary medicine have an important place in health care - leading to the concept that an integrative approach would have the most successful outcome for all involved.

Too often, we are guilty of deriving negative connotations from terms like *alternative* and *complementary*. Yet, according to Webster, the word alternative simply suggests "offering or exploring a choice." Webster's definition for complementary is "serving to fill out or complete" and "mutually supplying each other's lack."[1] In other words, complementary medicine is not necessarily meant to replace conventional care but rather to *complete* it. Health care providers are able to offer respectable, even optimal, choices to their patients once they become educated on sound alternative or complementary therapeutic options available as well as the purposes they serve within the health care system. Ultimately, a comprehensive approach to wellness will enhance the existing level of patient care.

Clearly, the value of complementary care has garnered an increased level of respect and support in the last decade. Recent statistics regarding the number of visits health care consumers make to practitioners of alternative therapies are impressive. In 1997, it was estimated that there were 386 million visits to alternative care practitioners.[2] That same year, the estimated annual out-of-pocket expenditures for alternative therapies were 34 billion dollars. To place things into perspective, that was five billion dollars more than what health care consumers spent on services provided by conventional physicians.[3] A 1998 *New England Journal of Medicine* study resulted in comparable figures regarding dollars spent by US consumers on alternative medicine.[4]

With health care consumers increasingly interested in natural solutions to their health needs, physicians in particular are seeking out and paying closer attention to effective alternatives. ThedaCare Hospitals of northeast Wisconsin have announced the beginning of an integrative approach to medicine by offering a new service known as ThedaCare Holistic Health. Referring to this new initiative, Dr. Dean Gruner, M.D., Chief Medical Officer of ThedaCare Hospitals, says, "ThedaCare Holistic Health offers an exciting opportunity to expand our view of healthcare beyond the hospital or doctor's office. Patients and providers need to feel comfortable talking about complementary and alternative treatments and products."[5] Similarly, Affinity Health Systems of northeast Wisconsin recognizes that "as consumer interest grows and data shows positive results, the less conventional medical therapies are becoming conventional practice."[6]

Understandably, there are alternative or complementary therapies that do not merit much consideration based on their lack of evidence to support a solid physiological rationale. At first, I questioned the degree to which hormones are involved in our lives and health, as well as the validity of the concept of correcting estrogen dominance by raising progesterone levels with natural progesterone. Yet, given the opportunity to learn the mechanisms behind estrogen dominance and natural progesterone therapy, the concepts become irrefutable. Therefore, I wish to convey that there *is* evidence behind these theories (both anecdotal as well as through scientific research) and it does make sense. History has proven itself. Hormone imbalance involving estrogen and progesterone can affect the human body on a variety of levels and prescribed synthetic hormones are not the answer they were once thought to be. Now more than ever, it is time to "think outside the box," or "bottle" if you will, when thinking of hormone therapy.

The "Prevention Principle"

When I started my nursing career, the trend in health care was said to be shifting from being "treatment oriented" to becoming more "prevention oriented." In fact, it was during this time of focusing on "health maintenance" that Health Maintenance Organizations (HMOs) became increasingly recognized and implemented. In reality, however, what I've witnessed over the years since then has been the use of more effective assessment skills and diagnostic tools which, while resulting in the ability to detect and diagnose diseases in earlier stages, have still not greatly impacted the ability to prevent them from occurring in the first place. As Dr. Nancy Snyderman, M.D., physician and chief medical correspondent for CBS puts it, "We (physicians) talk preventative stuff but we don't do it very well."[7] However, it would be worthwhile for prevention to become the primary focus of the medical community as the majority of illnesses treated in the United States stem from preventable causes. A 1993 report found in the *New England Journal of Medicine* stated that preventable illnesses account for almost 70 percent of all diseases and associated costs.[8] Some experts estimate that figure to be even higher.

With this in mind, in order to achieve a higher rate of disease prevention, one area worth focusing more attention on is educating people about confirmed as well as probable causes to common health concerns. We have seen how effective education can be in regards to the link between smoking and lung cancer. Rates of lung and oral cancer have declined steadily in recent years. In the same way, education regarding the widespread situation of estrogen dominance present among North American women today - the factors that cause it *and* the health conditions that are associated with it - could be equally effective. Furthermore, the strong relationship between prescribed synthetic hormones such as those found in hormone replacement or birth control medications and serious health concerns needs to be conveyed. Such substantial evidence exists to demonstrate these links that, with education, prevention could become a reality in more cases.

Believing wholeheartedly that prevention is where our focus needs to lie, I have made this book a comprehensive guide to how the pertinent issues surrounding the critical ways hormones – both endogenous and exogenous - relate to our health. I also describe the manner in which hormone balance affects our lives in ways that could transform the current state of health care to becoming more prevention-oriented. Respecting the importance of credible information and research, I have compiled my data from a variety of reputable sources.

Summary

Little by little, I foresee a transition about to take place in the medical world today as more health care professionals begin to recognize the significant role hormones play in our lives and health. Medical personnel are also starting to acknowledge there can be valid rationales surrounding the safety and efficacy of certain natural therapies. The benefits these therapies have to offer, in lieu of conventionally prescribed medications, are becoming increasingly recognized, sought after, and embraced. It is paramount that physicians and other health care providers consider it worthwhile to educate themselves and their patients regarding the roles hormones play in a variety of health situations, as well as the roles that less conventional treatments have in being regarded as sound, therapeutic options.

Thank you for taking advantage of this opportunity to learn more about hormone balance and how it affects our lives and health. It is exciting for me to share with you just a portion of the timely, pivotal, and "practice-changing" information I have accumulated these past several years. As health care constantly changes, and laypersons become more educated and interested in being personally involved in the decisions surrounding their health needs, a resource for obtaining current, credible information regarding these important issues can only serve to enhance the level of care provided. Without a doubt, improving the level of care given to our patients is the "shared goal" of all of us involved in the life-impacting profession of healthcare.

2

A Physician's Perspective

The following words are written by Robert Gottesman, M.D., a private practice physician in the Santa Ynez Valley, CA. He shares some insightful thoughts from a physician's perspective that many in the health care profession will find they can relate to. Special thanks to Dr. Gottesman for his permission to use this valuable column in my book!

A Progesterone Saga
By Robert Gottesman, M.D.

About four years ago, I picked up a small monograph in a bookstore entitled *"Natural Progesterone, The Multiple Roles of a Remarkable Hormone,"* by John Lee, M.D. It looked interesting so I bought it, took it home, and read it. As I read through it, I kept thinking to myself, "Why don't I know this information about natural progesterone?" I was puzzled and a bit distressed. I am a well-trained, University of Chicago physician with 25 years of practice. Why didn't I know about the antidepressant effects of progesterone, or the diuretic effects, or the incredible differences of progesterone, or that it is well absorbed transdermally, or that it can be used without estrogen to control menopausal symptoms? Dr. Lee was not talking about some flaky fringe therapy. He was talking about progesterone – a hormone that is produced in a woman's monthly cycle in more abundance than estrogen by a factor of ten! Arguably, progesterone could be considered the principal hormone of women. To be under informed about it is a serious oversight.

Somewhat frantically, because I knew that if Dr. Lee was correct then my medical "Weltanschauung" [philosophy] would be irrevocably altered, I reviewed all of the original references listed in the book's bibliography. If he was correct, it meant that our system of medical education and practice was flawed at a most basic level. Tearing through the literature, I discovered that, in fact, the data was there to support most of his positions. There weren't a tremendous amount of studies, but enough to realize that modern medicine was overlooking a very valuable therapeutic modality.

I also found substantial confusion in the literature. Numerous journal articles and books were obviously befuddled about the differences between progestins and progesterone. Frequently, I would find misstatements like this one out of *"Dr. Susan Love's Breast Book"*, "There is a new type of progesterone that has just come out" (page 208). (Obviously there is no such thing as a new progesterone, only a new progestin) Frequently, I found that concerns/side effects that are targeted at the progestins spill over to progesterone which then gets a negative spin.

Continuing my investigation, I started asking other physicians about progesterone. Somewhat to my relief, because I thought I might be the only one ignorant of this hormone, I discovered that they too were grossly under informed about it. Unfortunately, I found they were mostly disinterested, or not uncommonly a bit hostile to the idea of using transdermal progesterone. "If it works, it must be a placebo," was a typical response, or "I only listen to the data, show me the data" was another common retort.

Despite the critics, I gradually and cautiously began to incorporate the use of transdermal progesterone into my practice. I was concerned because its use was not the "standard of care" which is frequently a criterion for malpractice suits. Nevertheless, I persisted and came to clinically verify almost all of Dr. Lee's observations. And like him, I too, came to believe that progesterone was a remarkable hormone. I started giving public lectures on the subject. Women were incredibly appreciative. I felt a bit like some kind of a shaman who held secret knowledge, because I was helping women who had been struggling for years, sometimes decades, with estrogen dominance and were now almost miraculously responding to this "unknown" hormone.

And yet behind all of this I felt uneasy, like a kind of medical stranger. An army of traditional clinical practitioners seemed to be galloping along, broadcasting their HRT (hormone replacement therapy) recommendations, headstrong, confident, all the while blissfully ignoring the main hormone of half of the world's population. How strange it seemed and how difficult for me to reconcile. I lost a good deal of sleep over this and, as it turned out, some naivete about the industrial workings of modern medicine. I began to see a kind of assembly line conformity about HRT advice, a conformity that seemed to be encouraged and perpetuated by a powerful medical/pharmaceutical complex. Millions of women might be helped with the simple replacement of a natural hormone but were being denied this treatment through a combination of inertia, misinformation, conformity, habit, disinterest, and possibly even suppression. Prodigiously influential special interest groups can weigh in and determine what studies are going to be funded or if they get published. One senior Ph.D. researcher I know tried to have his original work on progesterone and apoptosis published. He had had numerous research articles published before. He submitted his innovative progesterone article to the journal with whom he had previously published, but it got rejected with the telltale rejoinder that if he repeated the research with Provera (medroxyprogesterone) then they would publish it.

Economic biases are deeply woven into the fabric of the medical/pharmaceutical complex. For example, 90% of HRT studies (over 300 to date) have been done with Premarin. But since Premarin is this peculiar cocktail of horse hormones, which includes small amounts of progesterone, we really don't know what we are saying about human hormone replacement therapy. Yet Premarin has become the standard for basing our advice to women about hormones. But is it estrone, or the horse-juice equilin or dihydroequilin that prevents osteoporosis, or is it the mixture? Or is it some of the trace hormones that are important? It is like the palace lie. The relative paucity of articles on progesterone is likely due to its unpatentability. Less money, less interest. This kind of informational brokering is insidious and pervasive.

I thought that within a few years, because of John Lee's work, the use of transdermal progesterone would become routine. Well, it is four years later, and I would hardly characterize its use as ubiquitous. There has been virtually no endorsement of it by the medical community. There is increasing use by women outside of the medical establishment, mostly due to John's tireless dedication. But, I am puzzled by the continued resistance. At these times, I imagine modern medicine to be like an orthodox religion with influential patrons. There are specialized high priests, cloistered researchers, white robes, and many who swear by sacred texts (like modern medical journals) and frown at the alternative heretics. As in Galileo's day, it seems that many won't look through the telescope to see if there are moons on Jupiter or not, they already know there can't be. If the word progesterone doesn't come from the "holy canon," then it can't be right. It would upset the established order of things.

In the case of progesterone, it only requires listening to the women to determine its salubrious effects. Of course, that's the rub too - many physicians don't listen. The "book" says nothing about giving progesterone to post-hysterectomy patients who take estrogen. But after listening to hundreds and hundreds of women who use progesterone in this situation, I find it impossible to deny its therapeutic utility. The brain has numerous progesterone receptors at various neural sites, and to ignore this fact and just prescribe estrogen (because "they don't have a uterus") is like a joke – were it not so tragic.

Thankfully, John Lee has "rediscovered" progesterone which, in this atmosphere rife with "leveraged information," is all the more remarkable. I, and the women that I treat, feel a great deal of gratitude toward him and his resourceful work. I admire his dedication and his consistent effort to expose the contradictions, misstatements, and inconsistencies that abound in our field. Incredibly, he has almost single-handedly trumped the entire medical/pharmaceutical dogma about HRT with the use of transdermal progesterone. It is clearly a more benign and effective form of treatment for menopausal symptoms and many situations of hormonal imbalance. I think it is likely that it will significantly contribute to breast cancer prevention. John Lee's work is at least 20 years ahead of everyone else in this domain. He has coined a new term in medical lexicon, "estrogen dominance." He gives lectures around the world, listens to thousands of troubled women, writes books and articles, and even maintains an excellent web page (johnleemd.com). In a word, I think his perspicacious ideas are, like the molecule he champions, remarkable.[1]

(Reprinted with permission by Robert Gottesman, M.D., private practice physician in the Santa Ynez Valley, CA)

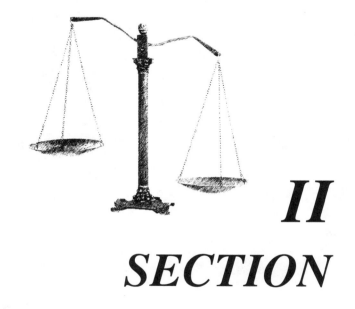

II
SECTION

Hormones and Hormone
Imbalance: An Overview

THREE 3

Progesterone, Progestins, & Natural Progesterone: Clearing Up the Confusion

Before going any further, allow me to define the terms *progesterone*, *progestins*, and *natural progesterone*. Clearly there is much confusion regarding the differences between the terms – specifically the substances they identify. While researching content for this book, I encountered numerous occasions whereby reputable medical journals used the term "progesterone" when actually referring to synthetic "progestins." With the medical profession misunderstanding the differences between these terms, and therefore the substances they describe, it is easy to understand how confusion is transferred to the general public. One contributing factor to this problem is that ever since progestins became recognized, pharmaceutical companies have errantly promoted them as "progesterone."

Despite enormous differences between progesterone and progestins, the terms are often used interchangeably. A main source of confusion stems from how progestins are commonly presumed to be included within a "class" of "progesterones" when no such class exists. Progesterone identifies one specific substance. To complicate matters even further, the terms used to identify progestins in European medical journals - *gestogens* and *progestogens* – are often confused with actual progesterone. Because of these errors, both endogenous progesterone (progesterone made within the body) and natural progesterone (plant derived) are often mistakenly thought to be "equivalents" of synthetic progestins in molecular make-up as well as in their actions on the body. [1]

One of the most extreme examples of how progesterone has been misinterpreted and misrepresented as the equivalent of progestins, was recently called to my attention. In some states the law requires companies that sell products containing "progesterone," such as natural progesterone cream, to issue a statement of warning on all of their labels. The warning they must print states, "Studies have shown that the use of progesterone may pose a risk to your health, consult your physician." The reality is, however, that the studies the warning was based on involved the use of *synthetic* progesterone constituents, otherwise known as progestins. Despite being referred to as "progesterone," progestins are entirely different than progesterone and are NOT found in natural progesterone products. Therefore, it is ludicrous that this type of warning should have to appear on the labels of anything other than what it is truly intended to caution against - the risks involved in the use of *progestins*. What makes this mandate most troubling is that it is purely the result of ignorance on the part of those in positions of authority who have implemented it.

Keeping the above examples in mind, the importance of understanding the differences between progesterone, progestins, and natural progesterone lies in that many are under the impression that a progestin such as Provera (medroxyprogesterone acetate) is the equivalent of endogenous and natural progesterone. A widely held belief is that they all share the same actions, side effects, and risk factors of which they most emphatically do not. Therefore, a proper understanding of each of these terms and the substances they identify is absolutely necessary.

The Power of Progesterone

The term *progesterone* identifies a single specific molecule. Although often mistaken for referring to a "class" of hormones (of which progestins are commonly thought to be included), it is simply a single hormone that has specific effects on the body. Progesterone is one of three primary sex hormones in women and men, manufactured in the body by the ovaries and in smaller amounts by the adrenals and testes.[2]

The value of progesterone stands alone. Progesterone is a "building block" for the other sex hormones as well as to the important adrenal cortical hormones essential for stress response, blood sugar and electrolyte balance, and blood pressure. Progesterone's other major functions include promoting and sustaining the development of a baby throughout gestation and providing a broad spectrum of intrinsic biological effects on just about every area of the body. This includes - but is not limited to – the manner in which progesterone can help the body utilize fat for energy, is a mild diuretic and a natural antidepressant, helps normalize zinc and copper levels essential for properly functioning neurotransmitters, and counteracts estrogenic effects by balancing estrogen and progesterone ratios.[3]

Progesterone plays a substantial role in a woman's life yet, progesterone is often a "forgotten hormone." According to Dr. Robert Gottesman, M.D., progesterone could be considered the principal hormone of women and to be under informed about its benefits is a serious oversight.[4] Progesterone levels fluctuate throughout one's lifetime because of intrinsic and extrinsic factors. Because progesterone is intricately involved in numerous important bodily functions, it is logical that a deficiency of progesterone significantly impacts the body on a variety of levels. As you are about to learn, this amazing hormone affects your life and health in countless ways!

The Problem with Progestins

The greatest difference between progestins and progesterone is the fact that progestins are *synthetic*. That is, they are molecularly altered in a laboratory to become patentable by drug companies and available by prescription only. It was only after Mayo Clinic's announcement in the mid-1970s that estrogen taken alone (referred to as "unopposed estrogen") was deemed toxic and carcinogenic, and the clinic's subsequent recommendation that progesterone should be taken alongside estrogen to prevent endometrial cancer, that progestins became widely utilized.[5]

Although natural progesterone (explained later in this chapter) was available and literature regarding its benefits existed, it was not a popular choice for drug companies to implement due to it being a non-patentable substance. Natural substances are not patentable and without a patent, drug companies cannot control who manufactures them. Therefore, because profits come largely from the sales of patented medicines, pharmaceutical companies were not interested in marketing natural progesterone. Instead, they decided to alter the molecular structure of progesterone to make it patentable, which led to the formulation and promotion of what we now recognize as progestins. By doing so, the pharmaceutical industry was able to gain and maintain control of this corner of the market and, as a result, the profits that accompany that market as well.

While progesterone is utilized in the process of making progestins, progestins are completely different from progesterone in appearance and action. To illustrate this point, I will use the example of petroleum crude oil which is refined to make mineral oil. Although petroleum crude oil is used to make everyday mineral oil, because of the transformation petroleum goes through to become mineral oil, it not only looks entirely different, it acts different as well. If you put mineral oil in your car instead of petroleum oil, your car will not run properly. Similarly, if you tinker with the molecular structure of progesterone to formulate progestins, it will take on an entirely different action in our bodies – usually in the form of unwanted side effects and risk factors. Furthermore, just as your own thyroid hormone is superior to its prescribed counterparts and the insulin your body manufactures is preferred to bovine or synthetic insulin, endogenous progesterone (progesterone made by the body) and natural progesterone (derived from plants) are superior to what synthetic progestins have to offer.

It is important to re-emphasize that the molecular structure of a *progestin* is entirely different from *endogenous* progesterone and *natural* progesterone. In the interest of becoming patentable, altering the molecular structure of progesterone to become a progestin radically changes its effects on the body - a feature our bodies are quick to recognize and react to. Unlike progesterone, progestins cannot be utilized as precursors to other hormones and are cumbersome for the body to break down and excrete.

Earlier in this chapter, I mentioned that certain states require specific warnings on labels of products that contain progestins because of their known risks. The bottom line is that progestins are not recognized as a fully compatible substance by the body and therefore have the potential to cause a host of undesirable side effects including cardiovascular complications, blood clots, insomnia, menstrual irregularities, depression, and masculinizing effects, and cancer. In fact, progestins are carcinogenic – that is, known to cause cancer. Back in the year 1988, progestins were listed by the federal Scientific Advisory Panel as a chemical demonstrating evidence of carcinogenicity based on evaluations conducted by the International Agency for the Research on Cancer and by the National Toxicology Program.[6]

According to the latest research, when progestins are combined with estrogen (as they often are in both birth control pills and combination HRT), they raise the risk of breast cancer even more than estrogen alone.[7] Despite its own inherent risks of causing cancer, it is ironic that progestins are commonly prescribed along with estrogen in the form of combination hormone therapy for menopausal women who still have their uterus to counteract estrogen's carcinogenic effects on endometrial tissue.

Natural Progesterone:
Complementary or Complimentary?

In addition to the human body, the hormone progesterone can also be derived from organic compounds found in plants. Through a series of processes known as hydrolyzation, the sapogenin molecule, most commonly obtained from the soybean or wild yam, can be converted into a form of progesterone *identical* in appearance (molecular structure) and action to endogenous progesterone, the progesterone normally produced by the ovaries at the time of ovulation.[8] Progesterone derived by this method constitutes U.S. Pharmacopoeia (USP) grade natural progesterone and is commonly based in a cream for transdermal absorption. USP grade natural progesterone possesses an "identical likeness" in molecular structure to endogenous progesterone. Therefore, plant-derived USP natural progesterone is indistinguishable from what the body produces. In other words, whether the body makes the hormone or if it is derived from plant sources, when the end molecule is identical, the body recognizes and utilizes it as the same hormone.

Clinical and scientific evidence is currently available, demonstrating the potential benefits of natural progesterone. Gynecologist, Dr. Ron Eaker, M.D. states there is evidence that natural progesterone cream is helpful for many menopausal symptoms. He indicates that data supporting this is beginning to appear. Two papers at the recent meeting of the World Congress on Fertility and Sterility documented significant improvement in hot flashes for women using progesterone cream versus a placebo. Dr. Eaker has used natural progesterone in his practice, specifically for hot flashes, and has seen reasonable improvement. Dr. Eaker also acknowledges many anecdotal reports of natural progesterone's effectiveness for PMS as well as for menopausal symptoms and expects more investigations to be forthcoming. [9]

Medical research regarding the efficacy of natural progesterone includes the results of a double-blind study performed by Drs. Helene Leonetti, Santo Longo, and James Anasti. Published in the medical journal *Obstetrics & Gynecology*, this study found significant improvement in hot flash symptoms among participants using transdermal natural progesterone.[10] In addition, a placebo-controlled double-blind study was also recently conducted to determine the effect topical progesterone cream has on the uterus lining, known as the endometrium, in postmenopausal women. Also published in the medical journal *Obstetrics & Gynecology*, this study demonstrated that natural progesterone cream protects the uterus from the negative effects of estrogen. Natural progesterone exerted a distinct anti-proliferative effect on the endometrium. In other words, it counteracted the estrogen-related accelerated growth of uterine lining cells.[11]

Data stemming from the latter study could prove extremely valuable on a variety of levels. For one thing, the fact that natural progesterone was shown to inhibit aberrant cell growth in the uterus could be useful in attempting to inhibit this type of cell growth in other areas of the body. Knowing how increased cellular proliferation in *any* tissue of the body heightens the chances of cancer developing, the use of natural progesterone to impede this process has potentially significant implications.

Also, this study strongly suggests that natural progesterone is capable of providing the same protective actions on the uterine lining progestins have demonstrated, only without the numerous risk factors and side effects associated with progestin use. In other words, despite the fact that progestins are associated with negative side effects, they are routinely prescribed in conjunction with estrogen ("combination HRT") in women with a uterus to protect the uterus from estrogen's negative effects that occur when it is taken alone. Based on the aforementioned study data, natural progesterone could be considered a safe and effective alternative to using synthetic progestins for this purpose. This is good news for physicians who are seeking safer alternatives to traditionally prescribed progestins and for women who are interested in using *natural* hormone therapy.

Natural progesterone in the form of a cream can be a viable option for women who want to safely and effectively treat or prevent hormone imbalance situations. These include symptoms and conditions that occur throughout a woman's lifetime. Gynecologists like Dr. J. Ron Eaker, M.D., have begun to make use of natural progesterone cream for patients with PMS and symptoms of menopause. Researchers involved in the study of natural progesterone cream's anti-proliferative effects on endometrial tissue write that transdermal progesterone cream has become a popular alternative to conventional hormone replacement therapy.[12] Physician and associate professor of the Obstetrical and Gynecological Department for Temple University, Dr. Helen Leonetti, M.D. states, "The most striking positive changes that I see when women start using progesterone cream are fewer mood swings, fewer hot flashes, and better sleep."[13]

Summary

It is essential to distinguish progesterone and natural progesterone from progestins. *Progesterone* is a single, specific molecule manufactured within the body. *Natural progesterone* is plant-derived and possesses an identical molecular configuration and action upon the body as endogenous progesterone. Finally, *progestins* are synthetic substances found in prescribed hormones including those used to formulate chemical contraceptives and hormone replacement medications. With this information in mind, it is my hope that a proper understanding of these terms and the substances they identify will prevail.

FOUR 4

Estrogen Dominance: The Concept & Causes

As designed by God, the human body functions optimally when a *balance* of factors such as hormones and electrolytes is maintained. For instance, just as the human heart can be sent into a dangerous arrhythmia from an electrolyte imbalance, an imbalance of the hormones, estrogen and progesterone - with estrogen being in excess relative to progesterone - is also capable of causing debilitating and life threatening conditions. Both women and men produce estrogen, progesterone, and testosterone, yet quantities vary between and within the sexes.

For many years, the World Health Organization (WHO) has been using saliva hormone assays to conduct hormone testing around the world.[1] Saliva testing has proven to be an accurate, convenient, and efficient method of testing for hormonal imbalance. Levels of biologically active, "unbound" hormones such as estrogen, progesterone, testosterone and corticosteroids show up most accurately in saliva, making saliva hormone assays the most precise, relevant, and convenient way to measure them.[2] In contrast, serum (blood) testing primarily identifies "bound hormones," those hormones that are encased in a special protein coating enabling them to be carried by the blood.

Dr. Peter Ellison of the Harvard Anthropology Department has been involved in assessing salivary hormone levels among various populations worldwide. From his research, we know that sex hormone levels are significantly different in women living in Westernized or more industrialized countries compared to those in less-industrialized civilizations. Interestingly, women of industrialized cultures such as North America have considerably higher levels of estrogen when compared to the estrogen levels in women of other, less industrialized populations.[3] In other words, estrogen is most often the dominant hormone relative to progesterone in North American women.

The situation whereby estrogen levels are in excess relative to progesterone levels in the body has been pegged as *estrogen dominance*. Estrogen dominance describes a condition that can occur in an environment of deficient, normal, or excessive estrogen when insufficient progesterone is available to balance estrogen's effect on the body. Therefore, estrogen dominance does not always refer to the presence of too much estrogen. It simply means that estrogen levels are in excess relative to progesterone - creating a hormone imbalance.

The significance and magnitude of estrogen dominance should not be overlooked. Current research indicates that estrogen dominance may lead to unfavorable health symptoms and even pose serious health risks. These symptoms and conditions will be explained in the chapters that follow but first it is important to understand how a situation of estrogen dominance may develop within the body.

Potential causes of estrogen dominance:

- **DIET**

    An imbalance of estrogen and progesterone may be attributed to hormones found in common food sources such as meat and dairy products.

For instance, the agricultural industry has known for years that they are able to have animals like cows and chickens achieve "market weight" faster by giving them estrogen rather than using feed alone. As a result, estrogen is passed along to consumers of these animal products and by-products, often contributing to estrogen excess within the body. In contrast, women who consume a steady diet of a variety of fresh vegetables with little or no meat and processed foods, are more likely to maintain hormone balance even through the menopause years. This results in a healthy libido, strong bones, and few or no symptoms of hot flashes. Most often, it is women residing in cultures other than North America who experience the benefits this type of diet has to offer.

- **ENVIRONMENTAL TOXINS**

Toxic estrogenic compounds (also known as xenoestrogens) include pollutants, pesticides, and petrochemical substances. The term "petrochemical substances" refers to petroleum-based derivatives such as mineral oil, present in everyday products including lotions, soaps, shampoos, cosmetics, perfumes, hair sprays, and room deodorizers. Due to their actions on the body - specifically how they fit into and occupy our estrogen receptors –

estrogenic compounds are capable of initiating some of the same physiological responses actual estrogens would cause. Therefore estrogenic compounds can contribute to estrogen dominant symptoms and conditions.

In March of 2001, federal health officials reported on a landmark study of environmental toxins in Americans, published in the *Journal of the American Medical Association*. This study was the first nationwide to measure levels of over 20 environmental toxins in human blood and urine, including those that were shown to disrupt normal hormone function and even cause birth defects. The study identified surprisingly high amounts of questionable chemicals found in everyday products like soaps, perfumes, and cosmetics through blood and urine tests of study participants. The resulting data has provided crucial information that could be used to pinpoint specific disease culprits.[4]

- **CHEMICAL CONTRACEPTIVES**

The birth control pill, along with other forms of chemical contraceptives, is widely prescribed today to treat a variety of conditions including acne, menstrual cramps, heavy menstrual bleeding, and endometriosis, in addition to preventing pregnancy. However, even in what are considered to be the "lowest doses" available, these drugs contain potent amounts of synthetic hormones (estrogens and progestins), capable of contributing to estrogen dominance. Be sure to read Chapter 26 for more on chemical contraceptives.

- **ESTROGEN REPLACEMENT THERAPY AND COMBINATION (ESTROGEN AND PROGESTIN) HORMONE REPLACEMENT THERAPY**

Contrary to popular belief, a woman's production of estrogen does not cease after menopause, but simply decreases by about 40 to 60 percent. This decrease is enough to halt the process of menstruation and the ability to conceive a child. Progesterone levels, on the other hand, drop to almost zero in most North American menopausal women.[5] This situation alone can result in estrogen dominance. That is why it is puzzling that the concept of restoring progesterone levels in menopausal women is frequently overlooked. Menopause continues to be viewed primarily as a disease of "estrogen deficiency." Prescribed commonly before, during, and after menopause, estrogen replacement therapy, along with estrogen and progestin (synthetic progesterone) replacement therapy, known as combination HRT, each consist of estrogens that are capable of contributing to an environment of estrogen dominance within a woman's body.

- **STRESS**

Because progesterone is a precursor ("building block") to cortisol and cortisol is released by the adrenals during times of stress, stress can deplete the body's storehouses of progesterone. This phenomenon results in decreased progesterone levels existing within the body. In other words, when progesterone is utilized in the production of the adrenal hormones for the stress response rather than being available to contribute to other hormone functions such as balancing estrogen, progesterone can become deficient, resulting in estrogen becoming the dominant hormone.[6] Therefore, the impact that emotional stress has on the physical body can be significant when it leads to estrogen dominant symptoms and conditions.

- **SEDENTARY LIFESTYLES**

The World Health Organization (WHO) has discovered that estrogen and progesterone levels tend to be more *balanced* in countries whose populations take part in more physical activity, including exercise and physical labor.[7] This discovery supports the theory that an inactive lifestyle can be a potential factor of estrogen excess or progesterone deficiency. Perhaps this is true because it is known that estrogen is stored in the fat cells of our bodies. One result of a more active lifestyle, including regular exercise, is the ability to maintain a healthier weight through the accumulation of more muscle tissue than fat tissue. It follows that less fat would mean less estrogen stores available to contribute to estrogen dominance.

Once I understood some of the reasons behind the widespread existence of estrogen dominance among industrialized populations like North America, I set out to learn the physiological truths explaining *how* this type of hormone imbalance is capable of contributing to many common health problems. In addition, I was eager to understand how this hormone imbalance could be corrected to alleviate or even prevent the onset of these symptoms and conditions - *naturally.*

We are a society that has become accustomed to a "quick fix" or "speedy solutions" to our problems. This mentality has transferred into the health care realm as well. It has become commonplace to focus on eliminating symptoms of a particular health problem without taking the time to correct the symptoms' underlying cause. For example, medications are readily prescribed for complaints ranging from depression, heavy periods, and painful menstrual cramping, to symptoms surrounding peri-menopause and inefficient thyroid functioning. This routine practice of eliminating symptoms without correcting the underlying etiology is known as "symptom-based treatment" of health problems.

While I understand the need to promptly eliminate symptoms such as pain or heavy bleeding in the short run, determining and treating the underlying etiology of a specific symptom or condition should ultimately prevail in the long run. For instance, when someone develops debilitating back pain, it is imperative to provide that person with prompt and adequate pain relief. Eventually though, it is prudent to begin the process of diagnosing the underlying cause of the back pain so that permanent healing and restoration can take place.

As a result of the research I have logged over the past several years, it has become clearly evident that there is a physiological process by which a number of common health concerns are related, at least in some part, to the hormone imbalance condition known as estrogen dominance. If a health concern has originated, even to a degree, from estrogen dominance, correcting the underlying hormone imbalance (estrogen excess relative to progesterone) by restoring progesterone levels along with eliminating harmful estrogenic sources is clearly worth exploring. It is an awesome realization to know that by staying educated, we have the ability to live with a body that functions as originally designed, with important hormones operating as intended – in balance and harmony!

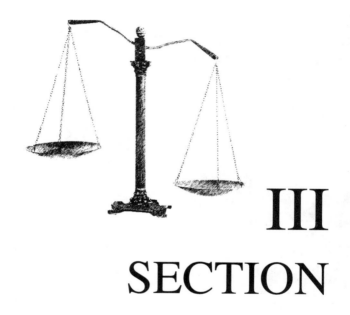

III
SECTION

The Hormone Factor:
Conditions & Symptoms
of Estrogen Dominance

FIVE   5

Solving the PMS Puzzle

From what I have witnessed, premenstrual syndrome (PMS) is one of the most common complaints among pre-menopausal women. Symptoms occur mostly in the two weeks prior to menstruation and sometimes for a day or two into menstruation. Common PMS symptoms range from water retention, breast tenderness, headaches, cramps, and fatigue to mood swings, irritability, depression, anxiety, and others. The causes of PMS are multi-factorial. Nutrition, exercise, stress, and hormones all play key roles. Treatment, therefore, has remained a challenge.

It would seem logical that women who experience PMS are at the childbearing age when progesterone levels should be normal. However, it is important to realize that estrogen dominance can occur even in the presence of adequate progesterone, if estrogen levels are in excess. So, while progesterone levels may register normal, estrogen dominance can still exist due to the various factors previously described such as diet, environmental toxins, stress, and prescribed synthetic hormones.

Interestingly, Margaret Smith, M.D., a well-respected hormone researcher and physician from Australia, reports that a colleague of hers recorded hormone levels in women for over 20 years. The results indicated that PMS consistently correlated with an imbalance of progesterone and estrogen levels - estrogen being the dominant hormone.[1] Dr. Smith has found that correcting this imbalance by increasing the body's progesterone levels with natural progesterone is a highly effective treatment for PMS.

Mood swings, depression, and irritability are just a few of the "classic" symptoms familiar to those who experience PMS. One cause of these symptoms can be attributed to an imbalance of copper and zinc levels since appropriate levels of these trace minerals are necessary for properly functioning neurotransmitters. Because estrogen can cause a protein in our blood to bind more readily to copper, an imbalance of copper and zinc can result. The imbalance between copper and zinc then manifests itself in moodiness, depression, and irritability.[2] Dr. Andrew Herzog, M.D., a neuroendocrinologist at Beth Israel Deaconess Medical Center in Boston, believes many women are depressed due to the imbalance of estrogen and progesterone.[3] Natural progesterone is capable of correcting this imbalance by restoring progesterone to its proper levels and, as a result, has been referred to as the "happy hormone." According to Dr. Herzog, progesterone exerts a calming effect.

The following is an anecdotal report given by a woman from Wisconsin regarding her recent experience with natural progesterone cream:

> I've been on the [progesterone] cream for just two months now and I actually got a "normal" period last week. I haven't had a "real" period for months due to being on the birth control pill in an effort to control bleeding. What a wonderful thing it is to have a normal period! Also, my husband and I can tell the difference in my mood swings since being on the cream. And, because I am having much more of a regular cycle, we have decided to try for another baby.

Medical professionals have been increasingly recommending the practice of raising the body's progesterone levels with natural progesterone for managing PMS symptoms because of the success experienced by patients who use it for this reason. In his book, *Holy Hormones!*, Dr. J. Ron Eaker, M.D., OB/GYN states that the use of natural progesterone is another popular approach to treating PMS. Dr. Eaker has used natural progesterone cream in his practice with success.[4] Dr. Jesse Hanley, M.D., medical director of Malibu Health Center and Malibu Health and Rehabilitation, uses natural progesterone cream as the basis of her treatment program for women experiencing PMS. Dr. Hanley has found that in women of all ages, the exclusive use of natural progesterone cream often alleviates the symptoms of PMS. Finally, Dr. John Lee, M.D., a Harvard Medical graduate, retired 30 year family practice physician, and world-renown author and lecturer on women's health issues, utilized natural progesterone cream in his medical practice for years with impressive results when treating patients with PMS. Closer to home, my own obstetrician/gynecologist shared with me the success experienced among his patients to whom he recommends natural progesterone cream specifically for the treatment of PMS. He indicated that patients report positive results without side effects.

Because estrogen levels rise with the initiation of the menstrual cycle, if there is a preexisting condition of estrogen dominance, the additional surge of estrogen would likely worsen PMS symptoms around this time of the month. Personally, I know countless women whose lives have been transformed since eradicating PMS symptoms by making positive lifestyle changes and restoring balance between estrogen and progesterone. Most commonly, women have reported noticeably decreased premenstrual cramping, as well as less moodiness and irritability. Many women, including myself, never used to have to check their calendars to know when their menstrual cycles were about to begin. The impending period was easily detected based solely on monthly symptoms. Now, however, those women must pay particularly close attention to the calendar to know when their monthly cycle is due as there is no longer an "advance warning system" in place!

SIX

6

"Not Tonight, Honey I Have a Headache"

Headaches and migraines seem to be affecting more people in recent years, even spurring the development of "headache clinics," stand-alone offices devoted primarily to the diagnosis and treatment of headaches and migraines. While there are many known causes of headaches and migraines, *estrogen dominance* is among those causes. In a recent national column written by Dr. Tedd Mitchell, M.D., director of Cooper Clinic's Wellness Program in Dallas, Texas, headaches were his "topic of the week." When describing possible causes of headaches, Dr. Mitchell pointed out that synthetic hormone replacement and birth control pills were culprits because of the estrogen they contain.[1] For years, the small inserts found inside the packaging of these prescription drugs have indicated headaches and migraines as potential side effects. In the next chapter, I describe a 23 year-old patient of mine who likely experienced headaches as a result of the estrogen contained in the birth control pill she was on.

There are a number of ways estrogen can contribute to the onset of headaches or migraines. One reason estrogen can initiate the onset of a headache or migraine is because estrogen reduces the vascular tone of blood vessels, resulting in a swelling effect of the vessel. Enlarged or swollen blood vessels are thought to be one cause of headaches and migraines.[2] Secondly, estrogen can lead to the onset of headaches by depleting magnesium levels in the body. Low magnesium levels can contribute to the arteries becoming more susceptible to spasm. This effect can be another cause of headaches and migraines.[3]

Estrogen-induced headaches can be alleviated or prevented by correcting the imbalance of estrogen and progesterone in the body. In addition to eliminating known factors contributing to estrogen dominance, by increasing levels of progesterone, natural progesterone is capable of offsetting estrogen's effects by re-establishing balance. Counteracting the effects of estrogen along with restoring hormone balance can offer headache relief as well as prevention in many cases. Natural progesterone used alone, to restore balance between estrogen and progesterone levels, or in combination with magnesium may be effective in preventing and alleviating headaches and migraines originating from the effects of estrogen dominance.

The "Low-down" on Unexplained Weight Gain & Other Symptoms of Low Thyroid

Without a doubt, hypothyroidism has become extremely common among women of all ages in recent years. Interference with the thyroid is one cause of hypothyroidism. Because estrogen and thyroid hormone have opposing actions, estrogen dominance can prevent the thyroid from functioning efficiently, resulting in symptoms of hypothyroidism - most commonly showing up in the form of weight gain, fatigue, depression, and low sexual libido.[1]

When describing the phenomenon of how estrogen can affect thyroid functioning, I am reminded of a gentleman I met who mistakenly took a prescription sleeping pill one morning instead of his blood pressure pill. Although there was nothing intrinsically wrong with his body or organs, he was clearly not functioning "normally" due to the sleep medication floating around his system for most of the day. A similar scenario can occur when too much estrogen versus progesterone inhabits the body and organs. The excess estrogen can inhibit the body's normal level of functioning in several ways – an under-active thyroid being one example.

Unexplained Weight Gain

Upon graduating from nursing school, I was employed on a cardiac step-down unit. It was on that unit that I met a physician who was starting his first year of medical practice. After a decade of practice, I asked this physician what he perceived to be the most challenging health concern facing his female patients. I found it interesting that after a brief pause, he responded with "weight control issues." He went on to explain that it never ceased to amaze him how many women struggle with their weight despite dieting and exercising. In Chapter Four, I pointed out the fact that the agricultural industry has known for years that by injecting livestock with estrogen they can be brought to "market weight" more quickly and easily than with feed alone. It should come as no surprise that the same effects can take place in humans with "estrogen excess." Whether from stress, our diet, by taking a form of prescribed synthetic hormone medication, or a combination of factors, we can also experience significant weight gain when estrogen is present in excessive amounts.

There are several ways estrogen dominance is capable of causing symptoms of an under-active thyroid, manifesting itself in the form of weight gain. The first way can be explained by recognizing that estrogen and thyroid hormone have opposing actions. Estrogen increases thyroid-binding proteins that cause the thyroid to function differently.[2] Whereas the thyroid facilitates the ability to metabolize or convert caloric intake into useful energy, estrogen "instructs" the body to convert caloric intake into "stored" energy in the form of fat.[3] Secondly, one of estrogen's actions on the body is that it tends to induce cellular replication wherever it resides.[4] In other words, just as estrogen can cause an accelerated growth (proliferation) of cells in endometrial (uterine) tissue (resulting in endometriosis, uterine fibroids, or even uterine cancer) and stimulate an overgrowth of fibrous tissue in the breasts (often leading to fibrocystic breast disease or breast cancer), it can also multiply fat cells. This often results in weight gain - despite one's best efforts to diet and exercise. Finally, because an excess of estrogen can cause fluid retention, and fluid retention contributes to weight gain, fluid retention is another way estrogen dominance can lead to weight control issues.[5]

Estrogen and Thyroid Problems – Coincidence or Correlation?

From my clinical experience as a registered nurse, I can attest to the increasing number of women who take both a form of exogenous estrogen (either the birth control pill or HRT) *and* a prescribed thyroid hormone medication such as Synthroid. In addition, I have witnessed a high incidence of women who shortly after starting a form of prescribed estrogen, experience symptoms typically associated with hypothyroidism. The scenario is all too common. The familiar saga begins when a woman starts taking estrogen in the form of the birth control pill or estrogen replacement therapy and eventually experiences symptoms of a low functioning thyroid – usually in the form of weight gain, depression, or fatigue. Sooner or later, she is given a prescription for thyroid hormone medication and may eventually require an increased dose due to the way estrogen steadily diminishes thyroid functioning. It seemed more than likely to me that there was a connection between these events as opposed to being coincidental yet I was unable to validate my suspicions with scientific data until recently.

In June of 2001, the *New England Journal of Medicine* published a study that provided reliable data supporting what I have observed in the clinical setting for years regarding estrogen's effects on the thyroid. The study demonstrated that women already on thyroid medication while taking estrogen often require *higher* doses of their thyroid medication due to estrogen's negative effects on the thyroid gland and binding globulin.

In addition, the study pointed out that many women who start out by taking only estrogen subsequently develop hypothyroidism, requiring pharmacological intervention with thyroid medication. The accompanying review article states, "In such women, hypothyroidism could occur sooner or be more severe because of the extra demand placed on the failing thyroid gland. Once they are being treated with thyroxine, these women may need a higher dose than they would if they were not taking the estrogen."[6] In other words, estrogen can actually induce the onset of hypothyroidism, necessitating a regimen of thyroid medication – at a potentially higher dose than what would normally be prescribed. I can't help but think that if estrogen dominance was detected and corrected in more cases, perhaps neither estrogen nor thyroid medication would be deemed necessary in the first place.

Could it really be that "failing thyroids" (quoting the aforementioned study) are just a normal part of a woman's life? Or have we just come to accept this phenomenon as "normal" because of how common it has become? The latter situation seems more likely. Because it is known that estrogen can diminish thyroid functioning, I seriously question if the majority of women currently taking prescriptions of both estrogen and thyroid hormone actually had an existing thyroid problem prior to taking the estrogen-based medication. The fact that it has become customary to treat "failing thyroids" by routinely prescribing thyroid medication correlates with the fact that symptom-based treatment has prevailed in recent years. However, instead of just raising thyroid hormone levels pharmacologically, it may be more beneficial to determine the cause of why so many women today are experiencing "failing thyroids."

Based on the number of women I encounter who are taking thyroid medications like Synthroid, I suspect that these drugs are close to the top in pharmaceutical sales.

Depression and Low Libido

In addition to weight gain, hypothyroidism can also manifest itself in the form of fatigue, depression, and diminished libido. What is often overlooked is that the onset of these symptoms may be related to a situation of estrogen dominance that has caused the thyroid to function inefficiently. Once again, symptom-based treatment commonly prevails.

Women who experience depression are often prescribed an antidepressant. However, those who are on antidepressants frequently experience unwanted side effects that may even exacerbate their depression. For example, by prescribing an SSRI (selective serotonin reuptake inhibitor) antidepressant like Prozac or Celexa to a person with low thyroid function who, as a result, may already be experiencing low libido, libido can be further diminished, because lowered libido is a side effect of these drugs. In other words, in addition to a woman's libido being adversely affected by a low functioning thyroid (perhaps due to estrogen's interference), libido is further taxed by the side effects from the antidepressant as well. As Dr. David Zava, Ph.D. puts it, women who have hypothyroidism and also take an SSRI antidepressant "get a 'double whammy' on their libido, and their sex lives for the most part are flatlined."[7]

It is possible then that the ultimate outcome of an even lowered sex drive could lead to heightened depressive symptoms if a lack of libido begins to negatively impact the physical component of marital relationships. Think about how a "vicious cycle" ensues whereby estrogen dominance results in low thyroid function; low thyroid function leads to symptoms of weight gain, fatigue, depression, and low sex drive; depression results in antidepressant use; antidepressant medication side effects lead to an even *lowered* sex drive; and this lowered sex drive exacerbates the depression. The frequency and significance of this self-perpetuating cycle cannot be overemphasized. Perhaps if women were able to prevent estrogen dominant situations entirely or were able to restore balance to their hormones, one or more of the recognized symptoms of hypothyroidism could be averted – a much better option than the opposite, yet all too common, self-perpetuating cycle described.

Briefly, I want to tell you about a patient of mine I will always remember. Rose (name changed to protect privacy) was only 23 years old and was scheduled for a preoperative consultation with me prior to undergoing a minor orthopedic surgical procedure. As I completed Rose's health history form, Rose indicated she was on the birth control pill, a thyroid hormone medication, an antidepressant, and a medication for migraine headaches.

As I transcribed her medications onto the form, Rose explained to me how she ended up with prescriptions for all four medications. She proceeded by telling me she had gotten married two years ago and started taking the birth control pill as a means of contraception. During the course of the following year, Rose accumulated a significant amount of weight, suffered several migraine headaches, and experienced mild depression. Rose informed her doctor and it was suggested that she be evaluated in several months to see if her condition changed. When things did not improve, Rose was prescribed Synthroid for what was determined to be an under-active thyroid. Rose took her thyroid medication and continued on the birth control pill, but was unable to lose weight despite dieting and exercising. Eventually, Rose felt as though her depression had worsened and she began experiencing more frequent headaches. Rose returned to her physician's office because of her persisting symptoms and was subsequently given prescriptions for an antidepressant as well as an injectable medication for her migraines.

It was three months later that Rose sat in my office and relayed her situation to me. Rose still had at least 20 pounds of excess weight to lose, she experienced migraine headaches several times a week, and she still described herself as being depressed. Furthermore, Rose expressed concern regarding the toll the medications were taking on her financially. Rose never realized the extent to which her symptoms coincided with the time she started taking the birth control pill two years ago until I brought it up to her. She did not recall anyone ever informing her that prescribed forms of hormones like those found in the birth control pill could cause weight gain, thyroid dysfunction, depression, and headaches. Nor did she remember ever reading the potential side effects listed on the package insert included with her birth control pill prescriptions.

Rose's experience is an unfortunate yet classic example of symptom-based treatment, proving it is wise to stay educated on health issues that concern you. Although I will never know for certain, knowing the symptoms and conditions of estrogen dominance, I have a strong hunch that Rose may have fared better with a work-up involving her estrogen and progesterone levels.

Restoring Balance, Restoring Function

It has been documented that many who have been plagued with symptoms of an under-active thyroid are able to restore normal thyroid function by restoring hormone balance. In addition to eliminating known exogenous sources of estrogen, using a properly formulated natural progesterone cream to counteract estrogen's actions can also be beneficial because estrogen can be stored in the body's fat cells for a number of years,

Natural, USP plant-based progesterone, is capable of re-directing the activity of estrogen, inhibiting many of estrogen's undesirable effects that interfere with thyroid functioning.[8] In fact, natural progesterone's actions are often likened to that of the thyroid. Natural progesterone is capable of facilitating thyroid hormone activity, promoting metabolism as well as energy. When Dr. John Lee, M.D. first started recommending natural progesterone to his patients experiencing menopausal symptoms, he noticed that those who were also taking thyroid medication were often able to reduce their dosages after several months. Eventually, a number of patients were able to discontinue their thyroid supplement completely. However, this should not be done without consulting your physician first.

Dr. Dean Raffelock is a chiropractor, diplomat in acupuncture and applied kinesiology, and a certified clinical nutritionist. Dr. Raffelock routinely assesses patients for estrogen dominant symptoms and recommends natural progesterone to normalize thyroid activity. He has found that balancing estrogen and progesterone levels often restores thyroid function while resolving other estrogen dominant symptoms as well. Furthermore, Dr. Raffelock states that using estrogen compounds like Premarin and some forms of birth control pills can raise T4 levels (an indicator of thyroid function), therefore "masking" or hiding a low thyroid problem.[9] This leads me to again emphasize the importance of detecting the reason symptoms have occurred in the first place in lieu of just eliminating them (symptom-based treatment), which can "mask" important underlying conditions. Perhaps by consistently identifying the underlying causes of the conditions and symptoms women experience, more women could avoid having to succumb to the inconvenience, expense, and unwanted side effects of taking an additional pill.

EIGHT 8

Fibromyalgia Facts

Perhaps you have noticed that an increasing number of friends, family members, and acquaintances are being diagnosed with symptoms of fibromyalgia. Its incidence has clearly risen in recent years. The pain experienced by those suffering from fibromyalgia is caused mainly by the state of chronic spasm the muscles are in. Instead of being supple, the muscle tissues become fibrotic or hardened due to spasm. According to Dr. Judy Gerstung, D.C., proper flow of blood to the muscle is impeded due to the chronic contracted state the muscles are in. As a result, oxygen and nutrients are prevented from entering into the tissue while toxins and lactic acid become trapped inside, leading to pain.[1]

Fibromyalgia can be diagnosed at any age and is often associated with fatigue, depression, fluid retention, joint tenderness, headaches, and insomnia in addition to classic muscle pain. Coincidentally or not, these symptoms closely mimic those experienced by people with estrogen excess or progesterone deficiency - estrogen dominance. It is also interesting to note that symptoms of fibromyalgia present themselves more often in *females* than in males. While it is unlikely that every woman with fibromyalgia is estrogen dominant, having estrogen dominance could certainly exacerbate fibromyalgia symptoms.

For many individuals, restoring hormone balance can help to relieve symptoms associated with fibromyalgia. In a recently recorded audiotape featuring Dr. Gerstung, accounts are given of people who have sought relief of this painful condition for years. By raising the body's levels of progesterone using a quality topical natural progesterone cream (see Appendix B), their symptoms have been virtually eradicated. Dr. Gerstung attributes the anti-spasmotic effect of natural progesterone as one of the methods fibromyalgia symptoms are relieved.[2] Years ago, natural progesterone was used to treat epileptic seizures during which the body undergoes a series of muscle spasms. This relaxing effect of the muscles is further demonstrated when specified dosages of progesterone are administered intravenously. Via this method, natural progesterone exhibits properties similar to those of a mild anesthetic.

It has been interesting to learn from several of my friends who have fibromyalgia that, after years of experimenting with a variety of conventional as well as alternative therapeutic modalities, natural progesterone has proven to be a helpful therapy for them. While it was the first time I had ever heard of such a therapy for fibromyalgia, these folks were already familiar with the value often found in it.

Estrogen: A Chronic Fatigue Factor

Chronic fatigue syndrome is another condition that has risen in incidence over recent years. As with fibromyalgia, chronic fatigue is most commonly diagnosed in females and can be related to estrogen dominance.

Estrogen dominance can contribute to chronic fatigue syndrome in various ways. One theory is best summarized as a "vicious cycle" that is sent into motion by stress. Stress can cause estrogen to become the dominant hormone in the body by depleting progesterone levels (refer to Chapter Four). The resulting situation of estrogen dominance then leads to additional stress caused by the consequential copper and zinc imbalance. An imbalance of copper and zinc can contribute to moodiness, irritability, and depression – all very fatiguing emotions. According to Dr. John Lee, M.D., "A woman who has been caught in this type of cycle for a few years will eventually find herself in a constant state of 'wired but tired', which will eventually result in dysfunctional adrenal glands, blood sugar imbalances, and debilitating fatigue that may be diagnosed as chronic fatigue syndrome."[1]

Another factor in how estrogen can contribute to symptoms of chronic fatigue involves *mitochondria*. Mitochondria can be characterized as the tiny "power plants" within each human cell that supply the cell with energy. Mitochondria convert energy from chemical bonds of glucose and other nutrients into a substance called adenosine triphosphate (ATP). ATP is used for energy by our bodies. In humans, mitochondria also break down a few chemical bonds of the cholesterol molecule to produce pregnenolone, which is used to produce progesterone. Unfortunately, mitochondria function less efficiently in the presence of estrogen dominance.[2] The excess estrogen interferes with the efficient functioning of mitochondria, resulting in not only less pregnenolone synthesis and therefore less progesterone, but also less energy.

Finally, recall from Chapter Seven (The "Low-Down" on Unexplained Weight Gain and other Symptoms of Low Thyroid) that estrogen and the thyroid hormone have opposing actions on the body. Research indicates that estrogen tends to inhibit thyroid function, resulting in symptoms of hypothyroidism such as weight gain, depression, low libido, and fatigue. Therefore, this phenomenon alone or in conjunction with other factors, may also contribute to symptoms of chronic fatigue in a number of individuals.

The exact cause of chronic fatigue syndrome may be difficult to pinpoint and is often multi-factorial. However, because of the numerous ways estrogen dominance can contribute to fatigue, many individuals affected with chronic fatigue find it helpful to identify and correct factors contributing to estrogen dominance by eliminating exogenous sources of estrogen or increasing progesterone levels with a regimen of natural progesterone therapy. Keeping in mind the importance of a good diet and regular exercise, restoring hormone balance can help to restore energy and stamina. An improved quality of life for those who have searched long for answers to and relief from their debilitating symptoms often results.

TEN   **10**

Fibrocystic Breast Facts

Fibrocystic breast disease is a concern for many women. Symptoms include breast swelling, tenderness, and lumps. Research indicates fibrocystic breasts are most commonly attributed to a disruption in the delicate balance of estrogen and progesterone – high estrogen levels relative to progesterone levels, otherwise known as estrogen dominance.

Fibrocystic changes in the breast are related to the way breast tissue responds to the hormones, estrogen and progesterone. Fibrocystic breast disease usually affects women between the ages of 30 and 50. In fact, the condition is less common after menopause because of a decrease in the amount of estrogen produced in the body. Of course, this does not apply to women who take chemical contraceptives or synthetic hormone replacement because of the estrogen they often contain. Stated simply, one of estrogen's inherent actions upon the body is to stimulate cell duplication – whether in fat tissue, endometrial tissue, or breast tissue. According to Dr. Charles W. Rice, Jr., the key to treating fibrocystic breasts is to avoid estrogen excess that stimulates the breast tissue to grow. Dr. Rice states, "Normal estrogen balance is essential."[1]

Recently, the *Journal of the American Medical Association* published a study that clearly demonstrates how prescribed synthetic hormones increase breast tissue density. The study also indicates how breast changes diminish with the cessation of synthetic hormone use.[2] In regards to the correlation between prescribed synthetic hormones and breast changes, Breast Health Specialist Nurse and Cancer Risk Nurse, Marguerite Goulet states, "It is alarming to see synthetic hormones so widely prescribed. One can see the changes in the mammogram of a woman who began to use hormone replacement therapy drugs."

Throughout the literature I reviewed on this subject, I read about health care professionals who have discovered how reestablishing hormone balance by eliminating known sources of exogenous estrogen and restoring the body's progesterone levels can resolve fibrocystic breast disease. It appears that once progesterone levels are restored and estrogen dominance is counteracted, breast tissue returns to normal, much like the above-mentioned study confirms. Dr. Helene Leonetti, M.D., a physician in private practice as well as associate professor of the Obstetrics and Gynecology department at Temple University states, "I always know which of my patients are using progesterone when I do a breast exam, because their breasts are soft as babies' 'tushes.' Only about one in 2000 women have fibrocysts that don't melt with progesterone."[3] Concurring with Dr. Leonetti's observations, I know women who routinely perform monthly self-breast exams that notice a dramatic difference in the state of their breast tissue by increasing progesterone levels naturally.

Finally, it is important to realize that experts believe some forms of fibrocystic breast disease increase a woman's risk for developing breast cancer. This is the result of the abnormal growth of glandular tissue that can become cancerous. Therefore, it is imperative to recognize that by maintaining hormone balance, fibrocystic breast disease can be effectively treated or prevented, possibly even averting the onset of certain types of breast cancer.

Miscarriage and Infertility Insights

The word progesterone literally means "*pro-gestation.*" It has been well established that progesterone is the essential female hormone for conception to take place and for survival of the baby to be maintained throughout the gestational period. During ovulation, progesterone levels quickly rise to prepare the uterine wall for implantation of the fertilized egg. In fact, women who are pregnant produce ten to fifteen times more progesterone than when not pregnant.[1]

Early miscarriages have become increasingly common in recent years. It is now estimated that about one-fourth of all pregnancies will result in miscarriage – half of them before the eighth week.[2] Only a small percent of miscarriages can be traced to a specific disease or genetic origin. "Luteal phase failure" is what is thought to be the cause of most early pregnancy losses. This means that as a result of a deficiency of progesterone during those first several weeks following fertilization, the fragile fetus is unable to remain viable.[3] Most of us have heard of women who require progesterone injections soon after conception in order to keep the baby alive those first weeks of gestation. Simply stated, without adequate levels of progesterone, the egg cannot mature. A failed pregnancy or miscarriage may then occur.

Another example of how inadequate progesterone levels can affect fertility is demonstrated by the prevalence of women with anovulatory cycles. It is becoming increasingly common for women of Westernized or industrialized countries to menstruate but *not* to produce an egg (ovulate) during their monthly cycle. In other words, there is an ample amount of estrogen to initiate menstruation, but due to inadequate progesterone levels, ovulation cannot take place. This situation whereby a woman routinely menstruates but does not ovulate is known as an *anovulatory cycle* and may indicate estrogen dominance. Anovulatory cycles eliminate any possibility for conception to occur and are often associated with symptoms of estrogen dominance such as weight gain, water retention, mood swings, fatigue, low libido, headaches, and sleep disturbances. Peri-menopausal women (women still several years away from menopause) who experience the symptoms of anovulatory cycles may be diagnosed as undergoing "early menopause" because of their menopausal-like symptoms. As a result, these women are often prescribed some form of HRT. Unfortunately, this course of action may only serve to exacerbate a preexisting, problematic situation of estrogen dominance.

Women who desire to become pregnant after being on chemical contraceptives may experience difficulty in conceiving. Swiss billionaire Fabio Bertarelli owns Serano Labs, manufacturer of most of the world's fertility drugs. In 1993, Mr. Bertarelli told the *Wall Street Journal*, "Our usual customers are women over 30 who have been taking birth control pills since they were teenagers or in their early twenties."[5] You see, our bodies tend to operate on the "use it or lose it" principle. With chemical contraceptives like the birth control pill, a woman's reproductive system is virtually shut down and sent into a type of pseudo-menopause for months or even years on end. Sadly, once a woman desires to become pregnant and chemical contraceptives are discontinued, the body often takes longer to resume normal functioning. In some cases, the body never returns to responding as originally designed. For more information on chemical contraceptives and infertility, please see Chapter 26.

Jerome H. Check, M.D. is a professor of obstetrics and gynecology and division head of Reproductive Endocrinology and Infertility at the University of Medicine and Dentistry of New Jersey/Robert Wood Johnson Medical School at Camden, as well as the medical and laboratory director for the Cooper Center of In Vitro Fertilization. Dr. Check, along with colleague Harriet G. Adelson, conducted a study involving women who had experienced infertility for a minimum of a year and a half. Published in the *International Journal of Fertility*, the results showed that 70 percent of the women conceived within six months while exclusively undergoing natural progesterone therapy. Dr. Check notes that too often physicians will treat an infertility problem with strong medication or even surgery without checking progesterone levels first. Dr. Check has found that for many women progesterone therapy is effective in helping them to become pregnant and to carry the child to term. He recommends that more drastic procedures be considered only after progesterone therapy is tried.[4]

While there are various causes of infertility and miscarriage, with the widespread prevalence of estrogen dominance among North American women today, it is of no surprise that infertility and miscarriage rates have skyrocketed in recent years. Unfortunately, due to a variety of factors, a woman's body is often deprived of a balance between the two primary sex hormones, estrogen and progesterone, and struggles to initiate or sustain the life of a much-wanted baby. If a woman wishes to learn more about using natural progesterone therapy for fertility purposes, Dr. John Lee's books are a valuable resource.

12

Progesterone & the Postpartum Depression Connection

Many times, the joy of a new baby is diminished by the onset of postpartum depression. Despite recent publicity, postpartum depression is still all too often unrecognized or dismissed, especially considering its potentially devastating consequences. It is estimated that of the approximately four million births occurring annually in our country, 40 percent are complicated by some degree of postpartum mood disorder.[1] At one end of the spectrum we see what is known as the "baby blues" while at the opposite end of the spectrum is the truly devastating condition known as "puerperal psychosis." Between these two extremes is what is typically labeled as "postpartum depression," a serious complication of childbirth. While depression is the major component, postpartum mood disorders can also be associated with symptoms like insomnia, headaches, mood swings, and loss of appetite. Postpartum depression may last for weeks or months, making life difficult for the new mother and her family.

In the previous chapter, I indicated how levels of progesterone rise significantly throughout the gestational period. This placenta-generated progesterone plays a crucial role in sustaining the life of the baby before birth. After 40 weeks of a constant, plentiful supply, upon delivery of the baby, progesterone levels plummet. This dramatic change in progesterone levels - from very high levels to significantly lower levels - can be a factor in the onset of postpartum depression in some women.

Research has reinforced the theory of hormone imbalance being involved with postpartum depression. A study published in the *British Medical Journal* indicated that women having the most dramatic fluctuations in progesterone levels prenatally versus postnatally had more of a tendency to develop postpartum depression.[2] In other words, women who were accustomed to the highest levels of progesterone before and during pregnancy, seemed to suffer most when levels dropped precipitously after delivering their babies. Due in part to how it influences the functioning of our neurotransmitters, progesterone is often referred to as the "happy hormone."

If identified early, preventing or alleviating symptoms of postpartum depression that are related to a drop in progesterone levels could be achieved by promptly supplementing with natural progesterone. Perhaps assessing progesterone levels in women a day or two after giving birth, especially in those with a history of depression, would be beneficial. In Dr. Katharina Dalton, M.D.'s *"Guide to Progesterone for Postnatal Depression,"* she states, "Progesterone is best-used at the completion of labor to prevent postnatal depression." By doing so, the underlying hormone imbalance is corrected as opposed to being "masked" with antidepressant drugs which can further complicate matters because of the undesirable side effects often associated with them.

For women at risk for postpartum depression who are taking oral contraceptives, Dr. Dalton warns, "Progestins are man-made oral substitutes for progesterone, and are present in all oral contraceptives. They are known to lower the blood progesterone level. Thus oral contraceptives should not be used in any woman at risk of, or currently suffering from, postnatal depression."[3]

13

THIRTEEN

Views on Vaginal Dryness & Low Libido

While there can be various causes of vaginal dryness and diminished libido - emotional as well as physical - hormone imbalance often plays a role. Think about the fact that progesterone is the hormone which begins to rise prior to the time of ovulation, peaking one week after ovulation.[1] When a woman ovulates, hormone-generated mucous is produced, increasing vaginal lubrication in order to effectively "snag the sperm." In addition, it is at this stage of the woman's cycle she may notice heightened libido. It is from the surge of progesterone, not estrogen, that libido is heightened.

In His perfectness, God designed our bodies to function this way in order to facilitate the procreation process – making it effective as well as enjoyable.

Birth control pills and other chemical contraceptives in the form of injections and patches are common contributing factors to vaginal dryness and a lowered sex drive because of how they inhibit essential hormone production by the ovaries to occur. With chemical contraceptive use, ovarian progesterone production within the body is essentially "shut down," leading to vaginal dryness and a lowered libido, in addition to the suppression of ovulation.

Recall that estrogen is generally still produced in respectable levels among North American women during the menopausal years, while progesterone levels approach the zero mark. Therefore, similar to women who take the birth control pill, menopausal women in North America registering very low progesterone levels often experience symptoms of vaginal dryness and diminished libido.

Restoring hormone balance can often help alleviate symptoms of vaginal dryness and also increase sex drive. For women who use chemical contraceptives, refraining from further use is often the first step. In addition, based on what we know about progesterone's actions upon the body, raising progesterone levels can also play a pivotal role in preventing or relieving symptoms of vaginal dryness and low libido. Many women experience the benefits of increased vaginal lubrication and heightened libido by restoring progesterone levels with natural progesterone. Both they and their husbands have experienced a renewed sense of enjoyment in this significant area of their relationship. Stasia Trivson, a national radio talk show producer and host, often shares the story of a woman she had introduced to natural progesterone. Upon encountering the woman and her spouse in public one day, her husband gleefully said, "Thanks for giving me 'my girl' back!"

FOURTEEN 14

Hysterectomy or Not to Be?

Dr. Stanley West, Chief of Reproductive Endocrinology and Infertility at St.Vincent's Hospital in New York, and author of *The Hysterectomy Hoax*, believes that, in most cases, a hysterectomy is not necessary unless a woman has cancer. Yet, well over half a million hysterectomies are performed annually.[1] Hysterectomies are often sought once traditional medicine fails to correct symptoms of heavy uterine bleeding, clotting, or painful fibroids. The unsuccessful treatment of endometriosis and ovarian cysts are other reasons women undergo hysterectomies. While natural therapies can often correct underlying conditions by facilitating the body's own healing processes, synthetic hormones usually only treat the symptoms themselves. As a result of the adverse affects women often experience from the high doses of synthetic hormones involved with this type of "treatment," hysterectomies are commonly sought as the next option.

While there certainly can be valid reasons for undergoing a hysterectomy, women should seriously evaluate the pros and cons as well as consider alternative treatment options. Furthermore, women should think twice about whether or not to have their ovaries removed in conjunction with the uterus. I am convinced each organ has an intended role in the body throughout one's lifetime. The role of the ovaries in females can be likened to the role of the testes in males. And while the ovaries continue to produce hormones that influence sexual libido as well as energy and stamina well after they are no longer needed for ovulation, women past the age of childbearing are often encouraged to give up their ovaries. It is usually considered justified because the incidence of ovarian cancer is rising. Yet we would never think of encouraging men who are no longer interested in having more children to have their testicles removed because of the increased incidence of testicular cancer!

Hysterectomies are often recommended for women who experience symptomatic uterine fibroids, growths inside the uterine walls. Incidentally, cases of both uterine fibroids and hysterectomies have increased greatly in recent years. Estrogen has been known for decades to cause cellular changes within the lining of the uterus, known as the *endometrium.* Therefore, it should come as no surprise that estrogen can play a role in the development of uterine fibroids and that, consequently, natural progesterone could bring about resolve by offsetting estrogen's proliferative effects on the uterus. Dr. John Lee, M.D. refers to uterine fibroids as another example of estrogen dominance and progesterone deficiency. He has found that when natural progesterone is supplemented from days 12 through 26 of the menstrual cycle, further growth of fibroids is often prevented and at times can even regress.[2]

Recently, there has been substantial research done in this area regarding the efficacy of natural progesterone by Drs. James Anasti, M.D., H.B. Leonetti, M.D., and K.J. Wilson, PhD. The medical journal *Obstetrics & Gynecology* published the results of their randomized study demonstrating the beneficial effects natural progesterone cream has on the uterine lining of postmenopausal women. The study concluded that topical application of natural progesterone cream has an anti-proliferative effect on the uterine lining.[3] In other words, natural progesterone is shown to inhibit abnormal cell growth and therefore could prevent aberrant cellular changes in the endometrium.

Heavy Bleeding and Clotting

Other conditions women may seek or be advised to undergo a hysterectomy for include heavy menstrual pain, bleeding, and/or clotting. Without a doubt, these are debilitating symptoms. The pain alone is difficult to handle and when associated with significant blood loss, fatigue can also result. I have a friend who at the age of 30 was scheduled for a hysterectomy for these very reasons. However, she decided to cancel it pending a course of natural progesterone therapy. It is now over a year later and she has noticed a dramatic improvement since her first month using natural progesterone cream. Here is her story:

> Ever since I began menstruating at the age of thirteen, I have had severe pain and heavy bleeding with my periods. My doctors placed me on several types of birth control pills, diets, vitamins, etc. to try to ease my discomfort and bleeding, but to no avail. I am

now thirty and was scheduled to have a hysterectomy on March 15, 2001. However, after hearing a discussion on women's health, I decided it would be irresponsible of me to go ahead with the surgery without trying natural progesterone to relieve my symptoms. My first period after using the natural progesterone cream for one month was entirely different from any other I ever had. Instead of lasting for seven days (with half of that time being very heavy), it lasted for just five days. While the first day of my period usually requires me to change my pad every hour (or else I need to change my wardrobe), the month I began the progesterone cream, I used just three feminine products the whole first day. I finally realized that my life does not have to be ruled by my cycle for weeks out of every month. The other thing is that I have struggled with depression and have taken antidepressants for about a year. I usually need to increase my dose for two weeks out of the month in order to stabilize my emotional and mental status. However, since supplementing with natural progesterone, I have not needed to increase my dose and have remained stable. I hope to eventually be able to wean off my antidepressant medication completely.

Ovarian Cysts

Ovarian cysts are another condition common among women today, oftentimes leading to an oophorectomy (the surgical removal of the ovaries) – usually in conjunction with a hysterectomy. During each monthly cycle, the cyst enlarges and stretches the surface membrane of the ovary.[4] As a result, ovarian cysts are often associated with mild to severe pain and sometimes bleeding. During pregnancy, when progesterone levels are very high, ovarian activity is inhibited. In an effort to "mimic" this situation, the conventional form of treatment for women whose cysts become symptomatic is usually suppression of ovulation via the use of progestins (*synthetic* progesterone) found in chemical contraceptives such as birth control pills, Depo-Provera injection, and Norplant. As a last resort, there is the option of surgery (an oophorectomy with or without a hysterectomy) to avoid any possibility of further cysts developing.

In lieu of taking synthetic progestins, an alternative treatment for ovarian cysts is attempting to raise levels of progesterone *naturally* through the use of natural progesterone therapy. Dr. John Lee's approach is directed at using natural progesterone from day 5 to 26 of the menstrual cycle in order to suppress normal FSH (follicule stimulating hormone), LH (luteinizing hormone), and estrogen production, allowing the ovary time to heal for several months.[5]

Endometriosis

Endometriosis involves the growth of endometrial tissue outside the uterus, usually extending into the peritoneal cavity. It can be described as a painful affliction whereby the tiny islets of the endometrium migrate outside the uterus and throughout the pelvic area often scattering and attaching themselves to the ovaries, fallopian tubes, bladder wall, intestinal wall, and abdominal cavity. With each monthly cycle, these islets of the endometrium increase in size, swell with blood, and bleed into the surrounding tissue causing a very painful and oftentimes debilitating inflammatory process.[6] The severe cramping and abdominal pain associated with endometriosis can be extremely difficult to endure. In addition, endometriosis can distort the reproductive anatomy in such way that it often contributes to infertility. While the exact cause of endometriosis remains unclear, it seems to be a disease known only since the twentieth century. Cases of this serious condition have *not* been documented by earlier physicians.[7]

Current conventional treatment of endometriosis is complicated and not always successful. One surgical approach involves the removal of tiny particles of endometrial tissue that have migrated throughout the pelvis and encompassing organs. Yet, this proves to be challenging and often only temporarily successful. Many of the islets are simply too small to remove completely. They eventually increase in size and the condition recurs. Hysterectomy with a bilateral oophorectomy, the surgical removal of the uterus and both ovaries, is aimed at eliminating areas of endometriosis while reducing or eradicating hormone levels as much as possible to avoid further episodes. However, this course of action results in the body undergoing a sudden state of menopause and is often associated with a host of unpleasant side effects.

It is promising to know that symptoms of endometriosis virtually disappear during pregnancy, despite often reappearing once the baby is delivered. As with ovarian cysts, this suggests that the sex hormones are involved and that quite likely the high progesterone levels present during pregnancy are an important factor.[8] Mainstream medicine has attempted to mimic a "pseudo-pregnancy" state by causing chronic anovulation (the absence of ovulation) using synthetic progesterone, *progestins*, usually in the form of birth control pills. Unfortunately, because the synthetic hormones found in these drugs are foreign to our bodies and high doses are needed to mimic a true pregnancy, they are often associated with numerous risk factors and side effects.

Dr. John Lee has successfully treated a number of women with endometriosis using natural progesterone based on the rationale that estrogen is what facilitates endometrial cell growth and the accumulation of blood vessels within the uterine lining. Natural progesterone is capable of limiting endometrial tissue buildup and preventing the monthly release of blood to the endometrial islets by counteracting the effects of estrogen. As a result, the monthly inflammatory process subsides, allowing the body's natural healing processes to take place and eventually restore the affected tissue back to its normal state.[9]

Recently, I received a compelling message from a woman regarding her experience using natural progesterone therapy for endometriosis. Here is her story:

> I went in for emergency surgery on May 31, 2001 for a complex ovarian cyst. The doctor planned on cleaning out more of my endometriosis in addition to draining the cyst. The cyst was twice the size of my uterus and the fallopian tube was completely stretched out. [However], after looking everywhere, she could find no trace of the endometriosis although I had a lot of it left after my last surgery. The doctor and the surgical staff were amazed! They knew that I refused to

take the Lupron, Danocrine, and Megace. I told the doctors that I had changed my diet, exercised when the pain wasn't too bad, and was on the Arbonne's PhytoProlief (progesterone cream). I was diagnosed with endometriosis on March 1, 2001, started the [progesterone] cream, and am "endometriosis-free" as of May 31, 2001!

Cervical Dysplasia

Cervical dysplasia defines the presence of abnormal or suspicious looking cells involving a woman's cervix that may be cancerous or pre-cancerous. Cervical dysplasia is often detected with annual PAP exams or through the process of evaluating symptoms of mid-cycle spotting or bleeding. Definitive diagnosis and treatment of cervical dysplasia often requires conization, an invasive surgical procedure involving the removal of the affected area of abnormal cells and surrounding tissues of the cervix.

While rarely a cause for hysterectomy, cervical dysplasia has become disturbingly common among women today. I have several friends that have undergone one or more procedures to treat this condition. A common thread among these women is that they all have a history of taking the birth control pill. In fact, in February of 2001, the medical journal *Gynecological Endocrinology* published the results of a study showing that women who use oral contraceptives have approximately a 30 percent greater risk of developing cervical dysplasia than women who do not use oral contraceptives.[10] On the contrary, natural progesterone has been documented to inhibit aberrant cell growth while promoting normal cell maturation.[11]

Post-Hysterectomy Hormone Replacement

Finally, for women who have already undergone a hysterectomy related surgery or who may do so in the future, I wish to address hormone replacement following these procedures. Recommendations usually differ depending on if a hysterectomy alone (the surgical removal of just the uterus) or a hysterectomy with an oophorectomy (surgical removal of the uterus with the ovaries) is performed.

The ovaries produce both estrogen and progesterone. Therefore, an abrupt loss of these hormones is imminent following a hysterectomy with an oophorectomy and hormone replacement is mostly a concern of women who have undergone this type of surgical procedure. Surprisingly though, even in women who have had hysterectomies where the ovaries have remained intact, literature indicates that in time, their ovaries often cease to produce hormones because of the disruption of blood supply stemming from the surgical removal of the uterus.[12] A woman's uterus and ovaries were designed to complement one another and function in unison. When one no longer exists or loses its ability to carry out its intended function, the other often eventually stops working as well. This demonstrates how each organ was designed to serve a specific purpose throughout one's lifetime and also how our bodies tend to operate on the "use it or lose it" principle. Therefore, even a woman with only her uterus removed (with ovaries still intact) could benefit from hormone restoration – natural progesterone and, with discretion, possibly estrogen. (Please see Chapter 27 - "The Estrogen Question.")

Ending Thoughts

Hysterectomies rank as one of the most common surgical procedures in the United States – unlike in other countries. Yet, hysterectomies can involve various physical and emotional implications. Thus, it is worth knowing that some of the reasons hysterectomies are performed in the first place can be attributed to hormone imbalance, such as estrogen dominance. Consequently, it may be beneficial to attempt to correct the underlying hormone imbalance prior to resorting to potent drugs or surgery. After all, it is considered standard practice in medicine to treat health problems using the most conservative methods first, and to rely on more drastic or invasive measures only after attempts with other options have proven unsuccessful. Finally, it is wise for women to consider replacing lost progesterone, in addition to possibly estrogen, following any hysterectomy-related surgery due to how levels are affected with these procedures.

FIFTE**15**

Gallbladder Grief

Gallbladder disease is the most common digestive disease in the United States, affecting over 20 million Americans. Gallbladder disease refers to inflammation, infection, stones, or obstruction of the gallbladder. Approximately one million new cases of gallbladder disease are diagnosed each year - half of which are surgically treated to remove gallstones or the gallbladder. Interestingly, statistics indicate that women are twice as likely as men to develop gallstones.[1] Therefore, it should come as no surprise that hormones and hormone imbalance may play a role in gallbladder problems.

It has been well documented that medications containing estrogen such as the birth control pill and hormone replacement therapy can contribute to gallbladder disorders. More than likely, this is largely the result of estrogen dominance. Other factors involving gallbladder disorders include diet, rapid weight loss, and obesity.

The gallbladder secretes and stores bile which is produced in the liver. Bile acts as a transporter for toxins and waste products being excreted by the body. Bile also breaks down fats that have been consumed, making them easily digested by the pancreatic enzyme, lipase. Bile is released from the gallbladder in response to food in the upper intestine (duodenum). Proper flow of bile is essential to one's health. Conditions or factors that slow or obstruct the flow of bile from the gallbladder result in gallbladder disease.

The Sphincter of Oddi is what controls the flow of bile into the duodenum by either constricting or dilating. The Sphincter of Oddi also controls the flow of essential digestive enzymes secreted by the pancreas.[2] The flow of bile and pancreatic secretions through the Sphincter of Oddi is dependent on the size of the sphincter opening and the viscosity of the secretions. If the sphincter is constricted, flow is impeded, causing bile and digestive enzymes to back up into the pancreatic duct. The emulsifying effect of the bile combined with the potent digestive pancreatic enzymes can cause serious damage to the pancreatic tissue, even leading to pancreatitis.[3]

Persons with an imbalance of estrogen relative to progesterone (estrogen dominance) may be more likely to experience a constricted Sphincter of Oddi. This is why the inserts accompanying prescription medications containing estrogen specifically warn women of an increased risk for gallbladder disease. Conversely, progesterone is known to promote relaxation of the sphincter, thus facilitating bile flow. Many women report improved digestion once they take steps to correct estrogen dominance. This includes eliminating known sources of exogenous estrogen while also raising progesterone levels. Keep in mind that excess estrogen can be harbored in the body for years and that natural progesterone can help balance the excess. Additional factors that promote a healthy digestive system include avoiding fried foods, sugar, and refined starches, drinking plenty of water, getting enough fiber, maintaining a proper body weight by avoiding overeating and rapid weight-loss diets, and chewing your food thoroughly.[4]

SIXTEEN **16**

Estrogen Dominance & Autoimmune Disorders: A Likely Link

It is thought that autoimmune disorders may be related to viral infections within susceptible people. The virus causes a production of antibodies that act against a protein component of the virus. The antibodies then attack similar proteins in certain body tissues. Autoimmune disorders are diagnosed by analyzing levels of and detecting the existence of specific antibodies.[1]

It is interesting that autoimmune diseases, such as lupus erythematosis, Hashimoto's thyroiditis, and others, occur primarily in the female population and are very much on the rise. Recent studies have indicated that women who use birth control pills or who are on HRT are more likely to be diagnosed with autoimmune disorders such as lupus.[2] It has been theorized that hormonal imbalance is involved, with estrogen dominance triggering the errant antibodies. I anticipate that scientific research establishing the relationship of hormones to autoimmune diseases will soon be brought to the forefront.

A conventional treatment for autoimmune diseases includes administering corticosteroids which are known to counteract an assault by one's own antibodies. Recall that progesterone is the primary precursor or building block of the adrenal corticosteroid hormones. Consequently, it has been theorized that if inadequate progesterone levels are present, restoring normal levels of progesterone would facilitate adequate corticosteroid production. Suppression of the autoimmune attack would likely follow. Dr. John Lee, M.D. has witnessed this phenomenon in his clinical practice.

17

The "Skinny" on Skin Conditions

Acne

Antibiotics have become a common form of treatment for acne. However, it is important to regard antibiotics as serious medications and to resort to their use only after exhausting more conservative therapeutic modalities, while also attempting to correct any underlying health condition. It is not uncommon for teens and adults to be on antibiotics for years solely to treat a problematic skin condition like acne. However, due in part to the widespread use of maintenance dose antibiotics over recent years, we are witnessing an increase in antibiotic resistant bacteria.

A recent article published in the *Joint Commission Journal on Quality Improvement*, pointed out that one-third to one-half of all antibiotic prescriptions are judged to be inappropriate or questionable. The authors of the article state, "The need to improve the use of antibiotic prescriptions has been designated as a high-priority area for slowing down the emergence of antibiotic resistance."[1] As a result of the indiscriminate use of anti-microbial agents, there are persons who develop a type of immunity to antibiotics and become virtually unresponsive to traditional first-line antibiotic therapy when treated for an infection. As you can imagine, this phenomenon can seriously affect the healing process as well as inhibit long-term recovery.

In addition, the use of antibiotics can sometimes inhibit the growth of "friendly bacteria," - those bacteria which actually protect against harmful bacteria. This phenomenon may lead to conditions of candida yeast overgrowth and others. The resulting situation can be extremely serious and even deadly if not detected and corrected promptly as the husband of a woman I know recently discovered when he experienced this first-hand. The fierce, systemic infection has taken him months to recover from.

The birth control pill is another drug commonly prescribed to improve skin clarity. There is even a birth control pill currently on the market that is targeted specifically for "great-looking skin." However, based on the research I have done, the birth control pill is another drug that should be used with great caution because of the potential for serious and even life-threatening side effects due to the large amounts of synthetic hormone it contains. For more on the birth control pill, please refer to Chapter 26, "The Problem With the Pill and Other Chemical Contraceptives."

Finally, I want to discuss the drug Accutane. Accutane is prescribed for severe cases of acne and has been the subject of much debate over the past several years. You may recall the highly publicized tragic incident involving Congressman Bart Stupak's son, BJ, who committed suicide during the spring of 2000 in Menominee, Michigan, an area of the Upper Peninsula I grew up in. The Stupak's are convinced that the acne medication, Accutane, is what ultimately led to their son's untimely death. FDA reports on the mood altering effects of Accutane have now linked numerous cases of suicide and hospitalization for depression to the drug within the past fifteen years.[2] Unfortunately, this is an extremely tragic example of how side effects of drugs can literally change or end lives.

While acne can occur in teens and adults, it is seen most frequently during puberty and adolescence when testosterone levels are high. It is interesting to know that acne is not found in men who have been castrated. Thus, androgens (testosterone and others) have been implicated as factors in the development of acne. When a woman in her late thirties or early forties develops acne, Dr. John Lee, M.D. suspects hormone imbalance - increased androgen production as the culprit. Dr. Lee's theory is that ovarian follicle depletion leads to progesterone deficiency resulting in increased adrenal production of androgens. When proper levels of progesterone are restored, androgen production is counteracted and the skin often clears. To quote Dr. Lee, "progesterone cream does wonders for acne."[3]

Rosacea, Psoriasis, Seborrhea, and Keratoses

Rosacea is another skin condition known to improve with the use of natural progesterone cream. Rosacea causes a rose-colored hue to the skin, particularly the facial area. Secondary symptoms include inflammation, flaking, and even itching. While the cause of rosacea is unknown, it is typically a chronic condition. Common forms of treatment include vitamin B12 injections and cortisone creams.[4] Dr. Lee has found that individuals who use topical progesterone cream on affected areas often report positive results.

Likewise, there are individuals who suffer with psoriasis, a chronic skin disease associated with red, scaly patches, seborrhea (a skin condition which causes flaking and itching), or keratoses (dry, hardened skin lesions which are thought by some to be potential precursors to skin cancer). Many of these individuals have found success with the direct application of progesterone cream. Some have even reported remissions after enduring these conditions for a number of years.[5]

Skin Summary

Please realize I am not attempting to minimize the magnitude that problematic skin can affect a person – physically and emotionally. The point I wish to make is simply that it may be wise to consider hormone imbalance and explore other avenues of treatment prior to resorting to long-term use of potent drugs like antibiotics, birth control pills, Accutane, or corticosteroids.

EIGHTEEN 18

Precocious Pubescence

A phenomenon sweeping our nation involves young girls reaching puberty at an earlier age than just a decade ago. A recent study published in the journal *Pediatrics* indicates that menses is established in a significant number of American girls by the age of eleven today.[1] It is not uncommon to hear of girls menstruating as early as the ages of even nine or ten. A woman who attended one of my seminars told me that her daughter began having periods when she was just ten years old. Another young woman I recently met told me that both she and her sister started menstruating at the age of nine. The notion of this happening led me to initiate a conversation with my mother regarding the ages at which she and her peers began to menstruate. Mom recalled that in the era she grew up in, most girls began their monthly cycle between the ages of fifteen and seventeen years old. Interesting!

In addition to an earlier onset of the menstrual cycle, the appearance of secondary sex characteristics, such as pubic hair and breasts, have become evident at an earlier age as well. Because of how widespread this phenomenon has become, we are beginning to accept these changes as "normal" steps in the maturation process of young girls. In fact, researchers are advising medical professionals to recognize them as part of a growing trend and to establish new "norms."

While some experts attribute these new "norms" to better nutrition, another theory involves increased exposure to estrogenic compounds. Estrogenic compounds are found in the air we breathe, the food we eat, and often in the products we use on our skin and bodies (See Chapter Four). They set the stage for an environment of estrogen dominance at a younger age. Dr. John Lee, M.D. shares this perspective:

My suspicion is that this early onset of puberty is caused by exposure to the xenoestrogens so prevalent in every part of our environment combined with diets sadly lacking in the whole foods that contain the protective phytoestrogens. The long-term consequences of early menstruation are a longer lifetime exposure to estrogen, with an increased risk of hormone-driven cancer such as breast and uterus cancer.[2]

Estrogen is the hormone that stimulates the initiation of the menstrual cycle as well as the development of female sex characteristics at puberty. Excess estrogen results in premature menses and an earlier presentation of secondary sex characteristics at puberty. Therefore, it follows that early puberty results in a longer lifetime exposure to estrogen, increasing the risk of cancer. Recall that one of the commonly known risk factors for developing breast cancer includes an early onset of menses due to the longer lifetime exposure to estrogen that goes along with it. Knowing these facts requires us to further investigate the issues surrounding this phenomenon. Clearly, the facts call for more attention and research.

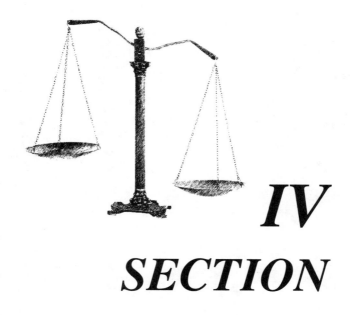

IV
SECTION

A Cancer
Growing Among Us

NINETEEN 19

Frightening Facts

In North America, cancer is probably the most dreaded of all diseases and with good reason. Despite enormous efforts to defeat cancer, the number of new cases of nearly every form of cancer has increased annually over the last century. According to the United States Bureau of Census, only 47 people out of every 100,000 died of cancer in 1900, making it the sixth leading cause of death at that time. Today, over three times that many people out of every 100,000 die from cancer, making it a leading cause of death, second only to heart disease.[1] More lives are lost each year to cancer than the total number of lives lost in the five wars the United States has fought the last century.[2]

What many of us may not realize is that other populations throughout the world do not exhibit as high an incidence of cancer, nor death rate from cancer, as North Americans do. However, as certain countries become more "Westernized," the number of deaths in those countries from cancer is increasing. For example, Japanese women traditionally experienced a very low rate of breast cancer, affecting only 3.9 women per 100,000 between 1955 and 1959. More recently, those numbers rose to 6.1 women per 100,000 and are still climbing. Furthermore, Japanese women who immigrate to the United States experience the same rate of breast cancer as American women after just two generations.[3]

In 1971, the United States made a commitment to advance in the area of cancer research following President Nixon's declaration, "The time has come in America when the same kind of concentrated effort that split the atom and took man to the moon should be turned toward conquering this dreaded disease." Since then, billions of dollars have been spent on researching cancer treatments, yet life spans for almost every form of adult cancer have stayed the same or increased. While working for some, conventional avenues of treatment in general have not proven to make great strides in curing cancer among the masses.[4]

Prevention is Key

In his article, *"The Thirty Year War: Have We Been Fighting Cancer the Wrong Way?,"* cancer researcher, Jerome Groopman, states, "Ever since 1971, when President Nixon declared war on cancer, oncologists and cancer patients have been caught in a cycle of euphoria and despair as the prospect of new treatments has given way to sober realities. The war on cancer turned out to be profoundly misconceived – both in its rhetoric and in its execution."[5]

After years of listening to predictions that do not live up to what they are cracked up to be, cancer patient-advocates like Fran Visco, president of the National Breast Cancer Coalition, are wary of researchers who exaggerate the so-called "successes" of preliminary findings and "cures." Referring to a recent meeting of cancer clinicians, Visco expressed disappointment at the way they interacted with the press. She explained her feelings by stating, "These clinical scientists receive media training and are scripted by their hospitals. There are so many agendas here: fame, patient referrals, fund-raising, pharmaceutical grants, academic advancement." Ellen Stoval, the president of the National Coalition for Cancer Survivorship, concurred with Visco's perceptions adding, "The headlines are dreadful." She referred to this type of sensationalism as "the pornography of cancer."[6]

Then there is the article by John C. Bailar III and Elaine Smith, which appeared in the *New England Journal of Medicine*. Bailar, who worked for the National Cancer Institute as a statistician studying trends in cancer incidence and outcomes, had become skeptical of the predictions surrounding the "war on cancer." Bailar and Smith's paper criticized the claims of so-called "advances" made in cancer treatments, instead proving there had actually been a steady increase in cancer deaths over several decades. The article ended with "we are losing the war against cancer."[7]

In other words, despite surgery, radiation therapy, chemotherapy, and all of the strides in medicine and technology, there has been no significant progress in the treatment of most adult cancers. The fact remains that two of every five North Americans will develop cancer and many will end up dying from it. Bailar and Smith are convinced that instead of directing funds and efforts on fighting this generation of cancers, energies should be focused on avoiding the emergence of tumors in future generations through prevention and early detection. In other words, Bailar and Smith believe that a shift in research emphasis, from the current focus on treatment to a new focus on prevention, is necessary to achieve substantial progress against cancer. I agree!

During my second year of nursing school, the curriculum included an explanation of how tumors develop. For the first time, I understood how both benign and malignant tumors develop as a result of cells proliferating (accelerating in growth) at a faster than normal rate in our bodies. Instead of a cell maturing normally, it regresses into a more primitive cell. This regression results in cancer. Therefore, wherever there is a high rate of cellular activity in the body, there is an increased risk that one or more of those cells will become cancerous. For instance, women who have fibrocystic breasts may be at greater risk of developing breast cancer because of the increased cell growth involved with that condition. Similarly, men with prostate enlargement may be more at risk for developing prostate cancer because of the high rate of cellular growth involved.

Although it makes sense that tumors - benign or cancerous - result from increased cellular activity in certain areas of the body, it seems to be almost too simple an explanation for such a serious diagnosis. For if we could somehow *halt* this process by which cells multiply at an aberrantly high rate, perhaps we could delay or even entirely prevent cancerous cells from emerging!

That is why it was fascinating to look at a remarkable placebo controlled, randomized, double blind study involving the exposure of estrogen and progesterone on breast cells. The multiplication rate of the cells exposed to estrogen surged dramatically, increasing their likelihood of becoming cancerous. In contrast, the rate of multiplication in selected cell lines was reduced to *normal* in the cells that were exposed to progesterone (not progestins).[8] By directing our focus to this kind of research, it would seem likely that cancer prevention could become a reality for many.

Corroborating research also demonstrates the beneficial effects natural transdermal progesterone has on specific bodily tissues. Appearing in a 2001 volume of the medical journal *Obstetrics & Gynecology*, a study designed to determine the effects of topical progesterone cream on the estrogen-stimulated endometrium (uterine tissue) of post-menopausal women, demonstrated that natural progesterone has an *anti-proliferative effect* on the endometrium.[9] In other words, unlike estrogen, natural progesterone inhibited the proliferation of aberrant cellular growth. Once again, findings like these could be the beginning of a breakthrough in discovering how preventing conditions that occur as a result of increased cellular proliferation such as endometriosis, fibroids, and cancer, can become a reality.

Every two years, a committee of scientists advises and updates the federal list of cancer-causing substances for the National Toxicology Program (NTP), a branch of the National Institutes of Health. In 1988, progestins were placed on this list because of their strong link to cancer. More recently, this panel of federal scientific advisors recommended that estrogen be placed on the nation's list of cancer-causing substances. On December 18, 2000 the NTP advisory committee voted that estrogens (the types used in post-menopausal HRT and birth control pills) be included on the list of cancer-causing substances because of their strong association to cancer.[10] Therefore, the issue of whether estrogens and progestins cause cancer is no longer a debatable subject. It is a well-established fact demonstrated through a consistent relationship that has endured the test of time.

Clearly, once the origin of a disease is recognized, prevention is well within reach. Based on what we know about the inherently unfavorable properties of estrogen and progestins, including their clear links to cancer, it would be wise for clinics, hospitals, and medical universities to be infiltrated with this information in order for it to become common knowledge. In the same respect, because of natural progesterone's inherently therapeutic properties, particularly its ability to counteract the carcinogenic effects of estrogens, natural progesterone warrants far more attention than it has been given so far in preventing and treating a variety of today's health concerns, including cancer.

20

Keeping Abreast of Breast Cancer

Breast cancer is the most common type of cancer treated in the United States. In the year 2000, there were about 185,000 reported cases of breast cancer among Americans. That number has almost *tripled* since 1960.[1] A woman's lifetime risk for developing breast cancer was one in 20 during the 1960s. Today, an American woman has a one in eight lifetime risk for developing breast cancer.[2] Could it be purely coincidental that the 1960s happened to be the decade *estrogen replacement therapy* became a "household name" *and* the "sexual revolution" began – leading to widespread usage of the birth control pill?

Clearly, we are not winning the war on breast cancer using common current approaches. Congress recently requested that the Government Accounting Office release its information on breast cancer. The accumulated findings, entitled *"Breast Cancer, 1971-1991: Prevention, Treatment, and Research,"* conclude that little progress has been made in preventing breast cancer or in reducing breast cancer mortality rates.[3] In fact, mortality rates are increasing. What I surmise from these facts is that *prevention* is the key component to waging war against this devastating disease.

Estrogen Versus Progesterone:
Effects on Breast Tissue

While there may be multiple factors involved in the onset of breast cancer, it is prudent to maintain hormone balance – avoiding a situation of estrogen excess or progesterone deficiency (estrogen dominance). A woman from my church recently informed me that her friend was diagnosed with an aggressive form of breast cancer at the age of 42. She was advised by her oncologist to read Dr. John Lee's books because of the crucial role estrogen dominance played in the onset of her breast cancer. Dr. John Lee, M.D., along with a rising number of other health care professionals, recognizes that the delicate balance of estrogen and progesterone is strongly involved in this devastating disease. Adequate progesterone levels are absolutely necessary to oppose the harmful effects of excess estrogen. Simply stated, estrogen is the hormone that *stimulates* aberrant cell growth while progesterone is the hormone that *inhibits* this action, allowing cells to mature normally.

While estrogen dominance can facilitate the growth of abnormal breast tissue, natural progesterone can bring cells back into a state of normalcy The protective benefits of progesterone were clearly demonstrated in a study published in the *American Journal of Epidemiolgy* by L.D. Cowans and colleagues from John Hopkins University. First, the estrogen and progesterone levels of the study participants were measured. The women were then put into test groups designed to monitor their susceptibility to cancer. The results indicated that breast cancer incidence was almost five and a half times greater in women who registered low progesterone levels. Furthermore, when the incidence of all types of cancer was analyzed, death rates from malignant tumors were ten times greater in women with progesterone deficiencies compared to women having normal progesterone levels.[4]

In 1995, a study published in the journal *Fertility and Sterility* was the first double blind, placebo controlled, randomized study using transdermal progesterone (*not* a progestin) and transdermal estrogen (estradiol) on pre-menopausal women scheduled for breast surgery. Study participants were divided into four groups and asked to apply a gel to their breasts daily for ten to thirteen days prior to surgery. Of the four groups, one received a placebo, one received progesterone, one received estrogen, and one received a combination of estrogen and progesterone. Blood tests and breast tissue from the operation were tested for hormone levels as well as rate of cell growth.

The study provided several interesting conclusions. The first finding of note was that both estrogen and progesterone are well absorbed through the skin (transdermally). After ten to thirteen days of transdermal hormone application, the concentration of hormone levels in the breast cells rose dramatically. Despite the fact that no measurable increase in hormone levels was detected in the serum (blood), levels increased significantly within the breast cells themselves. This substantiates that testing blood levels of progesterone is not useful in tracking actual progesterone absorption.

Secondly, the study illustrated that the women using the transdermal progesterone demonstrated dramatically reduced cell multiplication rates compared to the women in the other groups. The estrogen caused breast cell proliferation (accelerated cell growth) while progesterone significantly decreased cell proliferation rates. In terms of prevention, these are profound examples highlighting the drastically different actions estrogen and progesterone have on breast tissue.[5]

Breast cancer expert, Dr. David Zava, has also extensively researched hormone levels in breast tissue. Dr. Zava studied estrogen and progesterone levels in breast tissue specimens from several thousand women who had previously undergone mastectomies for breast cancer. These results, published in *Nutrition and Cancer* (1997), demonstrate a consistent deficiency in progesterone relative to estrogen (estrogen dominance) in the cancerous tissue examined.[6]

In addition, close to a dozen retrospective studies have demonstrated a longer disease-free or overall survival rate in women who have had breast cancer surgery in the early luteal phase of their menstrual cycle when progesterone is thought to be at its highest levels compared with surgery performed during the proliferative phase when progesterone levels are low. Published in a volume of the *Journal of Women's Health*, Dr. William Hrushesky of the Stratton VA Medical Center in Albany, New York reviewed this data and outlined in great detail numerous specific ways by which natural progesterone is capable of inhibiting breast cancer cell growth and metastases.[7]

Estrogen and Progesterone Receptors

Working in surgery for a number of years, I can tell you that it is routine for surgically removed breast tissue to be taken to the lab for testing of estrogen and progesterone receptors. Because the rationale for doing so can be a source of misunderstanding, I briefly want to explain the significance of estrogen and progesterone receptors found in breast cancer tissue. Hormones act by binding to their specific hormone receptors. Simply stated, if the receptors do not exist, the hormone cannot exert its effect. Dr. John Lee, M.D. explains, "You will not get a phone call if you do not have a telephone." Therefore, based on what we know about how estrogen is considered a cancer-causing agent, tissue testing positive for estrogen receptors could mean that estrogen was a major factor in contributing to that breast cancer.[8]

On the other hand, progesterone's actions are known to be inherently protective against breast cancer, yet it is capable of providing this protection only if the breast cells have progesterone receptors. In other words, referring to Dr. Lee's "phone" analogy again, *estrogen* would be the "wrong" message for the receptors to "hear" while *progesterone* would be the "right" one to "hear." Unfortunately, when progesterone receptors are detected in breast cancer tissue, a woman is often advised against using not only progestins, but natural progesterone as well.

Misunderstanding often occurs when those who advise against the use of natural progesterone either confuse natural progesterone with progestins (which you indeed would want to avoid) and/or are of the belief that simply because progesterone receptors are present, progesterone has imposed harm. However, once again, it is the action of the hormone on the receptor that is most important, not the fact that the receptor is simply present. It has been demonstrated time and time again that the actions of estrogen and progestins within the body have been found to be associated with an increased risk of developing cancer. Conversely, progesterone's actions are *protective*. Time and again, natural progesterone has demonstrated protective properties against the development of cancer.[9]

Traditional Risk Factors

Traditional risk factors of breast cancer include an early onset of menses, the late onset of menopause, a first pregnancy later in life or no pregnancy at all, and prescribed synthetic hormone use in the forms of birth control pills and hormone replacement medications. Upon close examination, the common thread among these risk factors is *a longer lifetime exposure to higher estrogen levels* in the body. In other words, an early onset of menses, a first pregnancy later in life or no pregnancy, a late onset of menopause, and the use of prescribed synthetic hormones (HRT or BCP) are all conditions that allow breast cells to be exposed to higher levels of estrogen for a longer period of time during a woman's life. Clearly, individuals with excessive levels of estrogen, either endogenously or from exogenous sources, face a heightened risk for developing breast cancer independently of all other risk factors.

Also consider the fact that stress is believed to be a factor in promoting the onset of illnesses and diseases, including breast cancer. One explanation could be because of the relationship between stress and estrogen dominance. Because the body uses progesterone to make cortisol and cortisol is released during stress, there is the potential for progesterone stores to become depleted with stress, resulting in estrogen becoming the dominant hormone. What this means is, stress can cause an environment of estrogen dominance, exposing the body to higher levels of estrogen and increasing the risk for cancer.

Scientists have begun to study the relationship between exposures to environmental toxins and breast cancer. The identification of environmental links to breast cancer immediately offers the potential for prevention. Extensive studies demonstrate clear causal relationships between health concerns and exposures to environmental toxins.[10] Sources of environmental exposure include food, air, water, soil, medications, and other consumer products. Over 90 chemical compounds have been implicated in causing the formation of mammary (breast) tumors in both males and females.[11]

Toxic agents that initiate or promote breast cancer act as carcinogens by disrupting normal hormone balance. They are referred to as *estrogenic compounds* and can be present in pollution, pesticides, plastics, skin care products, and pharmaceutical drugs. These toxins are broken down into carcinogenic forms of estrogen by the body. They biologically mimic estrogen and make human breast cancer cells grow in a laboratory environment.[12] Federal health officials recently released the findings of a landmark study on certain types of questionable chemicals Americans harbor in their bodies which were shown to alter hormone balance. It is well documented that many environmental toxins can accumulate in the body fat, take on the form of estrogen, and are carried by women in their breast tissue. Clearly, the potential exists for toxic estrogenic compounds to disrupt normal hormone balance, particularly in the vulnerable breast tissue.

Gene-Related Links of Estrogen to Breast Cancer

In their comprehensive report, "Estrogen and the Risk of Breast Cancer," published recently in a the *New England Journal of Medicine*, Drs. Mark Clemons and Paul Goss provide an extensive overview of the mechanisms by which estrogen causes breast cancer, right down to the level of DNA damage and genotoxicity.[13] Certain genes called *proto-oncogenes* start out as normal cells but may later develop into cancer. In other words, tumor formation may occur through the activation of proto-oncogenes.[14] The prefix "onco" literally means cancer.

Biologists have been investigating the actions of two genes identified as Bcl-2 and p53. Bcl-2 is a proto-oncogene while gene p53 identifies a gene that suppresses tumor formation (tumor suppressor gene). It has been well documented that proto-oncogene Bcl-2 production promotes breast, ovary, endometrial, and prostate cancer, as well as follicular B cell lymphoma. Conversely, tumor suppressor gene p53 inhibits Bcl-2 action, thus helping prevent cancer.[15]

In regards to the actions of estrogen and progesterone on these two genes, researchers B. Formby and T.S. Wiley discovered that when estradiol (a form of estrogen) is added to cancer cell cultures, in concentrations similar to those found in the body, the proto-oncogene Bcl-2 is activated, thus promoting cancer growth. With this information, at least one gene-related mechanism linking estrogen to cancer formation has been identified. This finding is further validated through additional research demonstrating how one of the pathways that metabolizes estradiol and estrone leads to a by-product that causes gene mutation and cancer (estrogen-3 and 4-quinone). In contrast, the addition of progesterone, in levels comparable with normal body levels, has been found to inhibit the proto-oncogene Bcl-2, while at the same time facilitating tumor suppressor gene p53, thereby halting cancer growth.[16] The implications of these findings in regards to cancer prevention are clearly evident but have yet to be given serious consideration.

Prescribed Synthetic Hormones and Breast Cancer

Evidence highlighting the risks of breast cancer involved with prescribed synthetic hormone use is growing. In particular the synthetic hormones found in hormone replacement therapy and birth control medications are strongly implicated in causing breast cancer.

Numerous studies have demonstrated the carcinogenic effects of estrogen as well as progestins on the breast. An in-depth report detailing the strong link between estrogen and breast cancer was published in a 2001 issue of the *New England Journal of Medicine*. The article states, "The connection between breast cancer and estrogen has been recognized for more than 100 years. Subsequent evidence has implicated both endogenous and exogenous estrogen in the pathogenesis of breast cancer."[17] Following this introductory statement, Dr. Mark Clemons and Paul Goss cite over 100 references illustrating their points. Even men who are treated with estrogen for prostate cancer or after transsexual surgery show an increased risk of developing breast cancer.

While estrogen alone is associated with a risk of breast cancer, research shows that the risk of breast cancer increases with *combined* hormone replacement therapy (estrogen and progestin medications like PremPro). This includes a 1989 study published in the *New England Journal of Medicine*[18] and a report appearing in the *Journal of the American Medical Association* in 2000. These studies demonstrate that taking an estrogen and progestin combination prescription is associated with an increased risk of breast cancer as a result of the addition of progestins.

The most recent study demonstrated that a woman's risk of being diagnosed with breast cancer increases with each year of prescribed synthetic hormone use. When compared to women not taking a synthetic hormone, women taking estrogen replacement alone faced a 20 percent increased risk of breast cancer. Women undergoing hormone replacement therapy with both estrogen and synthetic progestins (combination HRT) had a 40 percent higher risk of developing breast cancer.[19] It is ironic that progestins, which are routinely prescribed alongside estrogen to counteract estrogen's carcinogenic actions on the uterus, actually place women at a higher risk for developing breast cancer than even estrogen alone!

Another important study, conducted by Thomas Sellers of the Mayo Clinic Cancer Center, demonstrated that birth control pills, consisting of both estrogen and progestins, significantly raise the existing high risk of breast cancer among women with a strong family history of the disease. According to this study, published in the *Journal of the American Medical Association*, the risk of breast cancer *tripled* in users of the pill who had mothers and sisters with breast cancer. Furthermore, if at least five family members had breast or ovarian cancer, women on the pill faced an eleven-fold risk of acquiring breast cancer.[20]

Recently, I received a correspondence from Breast Health Specialist Nurse and Cancer Risk Nurse, Marguerite Goulet. This is what she had to say in regards to hormone replacement therapy and breast cancer:

> I work for a three-hospital health care system. I am overwhelmed with the number of women we see with breast cancer. We are observing increasing numbers of younger, pre-menopausal women diagnosed. We know that hormones are a factor to the development of breast cancer. That is why it is so alarming to see synthetic hormones so widely prescribed. It is offered as a solution to all of your health concerns as an aging woman by the vast majority of OB-GYNs, internal medicine, and family practice physicians here. One can see changes in the mammogram of a woman who began to use hormone replacement therapy drugs.

With such strong evidence linking prescribed synthetic hormones to breast cancer, it is disturbing that more education is not directed at making health care professionals aware of these facts. Two colleagues recently attended an all day women's health seminar geared toward health care professionals and shared the curriculum with me. Despite the evidence that exists, no mention was made of prescribed synthetic hormones among the fifteen breast cancer risk factors listed within the course outline.

Conclusion

For years I struggled to understand why the incidence of breast cancer has skyrocketed the past several decades. It only took coming to work on a regular basis, participating in more mastectomy surgeries, and conducting pre-op consultations to a greater number of women facing upcoming breast cancer surgery to realize that the incidence of breast cancer is nearing epidemic levels. Since doing this research, however, I have a much better understanding of why breast cancer rates are so high. Hormone imbalance is clearly a major factor. Interestingly, it seems that the breast cancer patients I have encountered in recent years often have a health history which includes synthetic hormone use

- in the form of birth control pills or prescribed hormone replacement. It seems to be more of a correlation than a coincidence.

We are clearly not winning the war on breast cancer today. There has been no significant change in mortality rates when figures are examined since the 1930's. Since the end of World War II, the recorded incidence of breast cancer has been steadily increasing. Although breast cancer research in the United States is primarily focused on early detection and treatment, the emphasis needs to be on *prevention*.

Just as we have made the risk factors of heart disease and lung cancer well known among the general public in recent years, it is our responsibility to do the same for breast cancer. Studies clearly demonstrate how regular exercise and diets high in fiber, vegetables, and fruits can offer protective benefits against breast cancer. Furthermore, because we are cognizant of specific hormonally related causes and risk factors of breast cancer, it is paramount that we concentrate our endeavors on breast cancer prevention through effective education on these and other factors. Utilizing this knowledge, breast cancer prevention can become a reality for more women.

21

Ovarian Cancer Makes the Headlines

"Estrogen Therapy Linked to Ovarian Cancer" was the headline that made front-page news across the nation on March 20, 2001. The headline appeared after the *Journal of the American Medical Association* published a study demonstrating that women who use supplemental estrogen after menopause for ten years or more double their risk of dying from ovarian cancer.[1] The study was conducted by epidemiologist Dr. Carmen Rodriguez and colleagues. An earlier study by Dr. Rodriguez along with the Emory University Medical School of

Public Health, and the American Cancer Society followed over 200,000 women for eight years. Dr. Rodriguez, lead study investigator, found that women who had previously used estrogen demonstrated a 23 percent increased risk of dying from ovarian cancer while current users had a 51 percent increased risk. In other words, a heightened risk for developing ovarian cancer persists even after a woman stops using the synthetic hormone. This finding was not influenced by any other factor such as age at menarche or menopause, family history, or body mass.[2]

Recall that high progesterone levels consistently correlate with providing protection against certain cancers, while low progesterone levels (usually resulting in a situation of estrogen dominance) often correlate with an increased risk. As with other types of cancer, this phenomenon has also been demonstrated in regards to ovarian cancer. Research has shown that postmenopausal women with either benign or malignant ovarian tumors often register *low* progesterone levels prior to surgery. In addition, it is also interesting that the more full-term pregnancies a woman has had, the less her risk of ovarian cancer appears to be.[3] Again, progesterone literally means "pro-gestation" because, during pregnancy, progesterone levels rise significantly. This knowledge contributes to an increased understanding of the protective and even preventative actions progesterone has on the body.

Ovarian cancer is recognized as a hormone related cancer. While still only fifth in cancer fatalities among women, ovarian cancer is on the rise. According to the American Cancer Society, over 25,000 women will be diagnosed with ovarian cancer this year.[4] Ovarian cancer is associated with a particularly high death rate because it is difficult to detect in its early stages when it is most curable. Most ovarian cancer is discovered in menopausal women and is of particular concern due to the fact that when diagnosed, the cancer is likely to have already metastasized.

The women I have known personally who have been diagnosed with ovarian cancer all happened to be taking prescription hormone replacement up until the time of their diagnosis. Time and again, HRT has been implicated in increasing the risk of ovarian cancer. According to a statement made in the *Journal of the American Medical Association*, case-control studies assessing ovarian cancer risk with five or more years of HRT use have consistently reported an increased risk.[5] Rather than chalk it up to coincidence, the facts support the relationship of ovarian cancer to hormone imbalance and prescription hormone use. Because ovarian cancer risk factors have been indentified, with education, prevention becomes possible.

22

The Problematic Prostate

The dramatic rise in prostate cancer over the past two decades has just about equaled the rise in female breast cancer. Prostate cancer is the second most prevalent form of cancer in the United States, breast cancer being the first. Based on data from the *U.S. Bureau of Vital Statistics and Cancer: A Journal for Clinicians*, the number of reported cases of prostate cancer in the year 2000 rose to 180,400 which is an increase of over five times the number of cases reported since 1971.[1]

In embryonic stages, the male prostate is equivalent in genetic make up to the uterus in females. Therefore, it is theorized that what is known about cancer of the uterus could also be applicable to cancer of the prostate. For decades estrogen has been widely recognized as the primary cause of uterine cancer. Because men produce estrogen, progesterone, and testosterone, and testosterone levels decline as men age, estrogen can ultimately end up as the dominant hormone in middle-aged and older males. And knowing estrogen's effects on the uterus cause increased cellular proliferation of the uterine tissue, estrogen dominance may very well contribute to increased prostatic tissue growth in males.

Without a doubt, men are vulnerable to many of the same factors known to cause estrogen dominance in women including stress, environmental factors, and diet. Furthermore, if testosterone caused prostate cancer, as is commonly theorized, males in their teens and twenties would be routinely dying from prostate cancer, because *these* are the ages testosterone levels are at their highest. While testosterone dominates in younger men, levels decrease as men age. Again, this could be a factor in estrogen becoming the dominant hormone in middle-aged and older men – the age group most affected by prostate cancer.

For years Dr. John Lee M.D. has recommended the use of natural progesterone to treat a variety of hormone related health conditions in women. Eventually, the spouses of some of these women began using natural progesterone to increase bone density and as a result, their prostate conditions improved. It was not long ago that I was informed about a gentleman who was being treated at Mayo Clinic for prostate cancer that had already metastasized to his bone. The man began using his wife's progesterone cream for his bones and after six months returned to the Mayo Clinic for tests. His test results indicated a significant improvement in the condition of his bone and PSA level.

Clearly, an increasing number of medical professionals, including Dr. Jesse Hanley M.D., medical director of Malibu Health Center and Malibu Health and Rehabilitation, believe that estrogen dominance is a major factor in the cause of prostate enlargement and prostate carcinoma. Other physicians are also convinced that prostate cancer may be associated with estrogen dominance and that there are benefits found in natural progesterone. Dr. Peter Eckhart, M.D. of Woodland Park, Colorado, reports on a patient of his who had an aggressive form of prostate cancer with a PSA (prostate specific antigen) level of sixteen. After six months of natural progesterone therapy, his PSA level dropped to less than one. A follow-up blood test several months later indicated an even lower PSA level.[2] Although more research is needed, preliminary evidence indicates that natural progesterone may play a pivotal role in preventing and treating prostate disease by counteracting estrogen's action of promoting abnormal cell growth in the prostate gland.

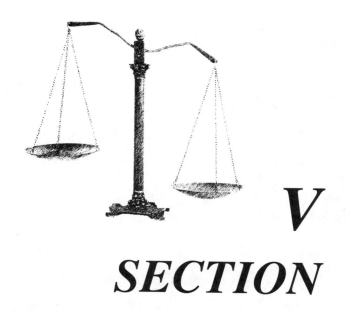

V
SECTION

A Message
About Menopause

23

"Menopause 101"

While menopause should be anticipated as the beginning of the "golden years," more often it is approaced with a sense of impending doom. Clinically defined, menopause refers to the time in a woman's life when she experiences permanent cessation of menstruation, in which the cyclical shedding of the uterine lining ceases and the monthly release of eggs stops. This phase of a woman's life usually takes place between the ages of 45 and 60.[1] Some women experience an earlier onset of menopause as a result of illness or the surgical removal of the uterus or ovaries (hysterectomy or oophorectomy).

While estrogen levels decrease at menopause, dismissed is the fact that estrogen is still being produced. The truth is that in North American women, estrogen levels drop merely 40-60 percent at menopause, while progesterone levels plunge to nearly zero.[2] Dr. Jerilynn Prior, researcher and professor of endocrinology at the University of Columbia in Vancouver, points out that when progesterone levels drop to almost zero, an imbalance of estrogen and progesterone often occurs, leading to the hormone imbalance condition known as estrogen dominance.[3] Contrary to popular belief, it is not always low estrogen that is to blame for menopausal symptoms, but rather estrogen dominance. In addition, as illustrated throughout this book, estrogen dominance can also contribute to other very serious health problems, including cancer.

According to the highly regarded *Novak's Textbook on Gynecology* (11th edition, Willians & Wilkins, 1987), while menopausal women do experience decreased levels of estrogen, estrogen is not negligible or absent but rather *sufficient* to support normal body functions during this stage of a woman's life.[4] Therefore, putting the blame of menopausal symptoms or other health concerns on estrogen deficiency is often not validated. With estrogen-based hormone replacement therapy, estrogen made and stored by fat cells, and environmental estrogenic exposures, estrogen dominance is almost a given.[5]

In addition, estrogen dominance or progesterone deficiency at menopause often occurs because of lifestyle differences, including dietary factors, among women of more industrialized countries such as the United States, unlike in women of less industrialized countries. Over 5000 plants manufacture sterols that are known to be progestogenic. According to the book, *Modern Pharmacognosy*, sources of dietary progesterone inclulde yeast, rice, wheat, cabbage, and potatoes.[6] Unlike women of North America, the majority of women in less industrialized cultures are able to maintain their sex drive, prevent osteoporosis, and float through menopause uneventfully due in part to diets consisting of an abundance of phyto-progesterones from a variety of fresh vegetables and little or no processed foods.[7]

Restoring Hormone Balance at Menopause

The ovaries are responsible for the primary production of both estrogen and progesterone. As women approach menopause the production of these hormones declines. Conditions including hot flashes, sleep disorders, mood swings, anxiety, depression, vaginal dryness, loss of libido, osteoporosis, and even heart disease are commonly associated with the onset of menopause in women of North America. For the most part, a decrease in estrogen is blamed for many of the symptoms associated with menopause, while the more precipitous decline in progesterone levels during the menopause years is often overlooked. Keep in mind again though, that not only do the majority of women in non-industrialized countries have healthy ovaries which produce sufficient progesterone, but their diets consist of a plentiful supply of progestogenic substaces helping to maintain sex drive, promote strong bones, and make the passage through menopause uneventful and symptom-free.

Because the ovaries are responsible for the production of both estrogen and progesterone, it is confusing as to why only estrogen is the focus of hormone replacement with menopause or a hysterectomy. Progesterone supplementation is often overlooked, except when a woman still has her uterus. If a woman still has her uterus, progesterone is prescribed usually in the form of progestins and in combination with estrogen to counteract estrogen's carcinogenic effects on the uterus. Unfortunately, the practice of considering progesterone only in women with intact uteri does not address the fact that progesterone's role in the body encompasses a number of valuable functions throughout a woman's lifetime - not only to protect the uterus from harmful estrogenic effects. The other functions of progesterone are hindered by any decrease in progesterone production by the ovaries – whether due to a gradual onset of a natural menopause or an abrupt surgical onset (hysterectomy and/or oophorectomy) – and must not be overlooked.

When gynecological surgery has taken place, the replacement of hormones is usually dependent on whether the surgical procedure involves a hysterectomy alone (surgical removal of just the uterus) or a hysterectomy with an oophorectomy (surgical removal of the uterus with the ovaries). Because the ovaries produce both estrogen *and* progesterone, and an abrupt loss of these hormones is imminent following a hysterectomy with an oophorectomy, the question of hormone replacement is mostly a concern of women who no longer have their ovaries. It should be known, however, that even in women who have had hysterectomies where the ovaries remain intact, literature indicates that in time, their ovaries often cease to produce hormones due to the interruption of blood supply stemming from the surgical removal of the uterus.[8] Because the uterus and ovaries were designed to complement one another and work in unison, when one no longer exists or is functioning, the other often eventually stops working as well. Therefore, even a woman with only her uterus gone (with ovaries still intact) would more than likely benefit from hormone supplementation by means of natural progesterone and, if necessary, a form of estrogen.

Progesterone is valuable. Therefore, restoring progesterone levels should be considered whether or not a woman has undergone a natural or a surgical menopause. With both situations, the potential for estrogen dominance exists. In addition, one of progesterone's properties is that it heightens the sensitivity of the estrogen receptors within the body. Knowing that the body makes some estrogen in the fat cells, if the sensitivity of the estrogen receptors is raised, then what estrogen is present at the time of menopause may be enough.

The notion that progesterone supplementation need not take place unless a uterus is involved needs to be re-thought and re-taught. Furthermore, it would be wise for health care providers to consider the benefits of replacing lost progesterone using *natural* progesterone as opposed to its risky, carcinogenic counterpart, progestins.

History of HRT

In the 1960s, estrogen replacement therapy became widely acknowledged as the cure to the "evils" of menopause. A 1964 issue of *Newsweek* carried a story entitled "No More Menopause" reported on the work of Dr. Robert A. Wilson who had been studying menopause. The story's theme involved the idea that menopausal symptoms occurred as a result of a lack of estrogen. Ayerst, a pharmaceutical manufacturer, took advantage of the opportunity to develop a prescribed form of estrogen, known as Premarin, for women experiencing the unpleasant effects of menopause.[9]

Premarin, the acronym for PREgnant MAre urINe, is made with the urine from pregnant mares. Premarin contains a variety of estrogens unfamiliar to the human body which is not surprising considering the fact that they are derived from horses. Among other things, what is extremely troubling about Premarin is the inhumane treatment suffered by the pregnant mares and their foals which supply the hormones used in its manufacturing, especially when alternatives exist. Nonetheless, Ayerst, along with Dr. Wilson, launched a large promotional campaign extolling synthetic estrogen for the treatment of menopausal symptoms.[10]

Today, Premarin is one of the most widely prescribed drugs in the United States, making it among the most profitable for the pharmaceutical company now known as Wyeth-Ayerst Pharmaceuticals. Because most women continue to produce respectable levels of estrogen during the menopause years, only a minority of menopausal women are truly considered "estrogen deficient." Therefore, it is puzzling to see the routine practice of prescribing additional estrogen in unnatural forms.

About a decade after its inception, the dark side of prescribed estrogen replacement began to emerge. In the mid–1970s, it was announced that estrogen replacement therapy by itself (unopposed) significantly increased the risk of cancer. This announcement led to making estrogen available in a lower dose (0.625mg) than the traditionally prescribed dosages of 1.25mg or even 2.50mg.[11]

With the evidence that estrogen taken alone is toxic and a known cause of cancer, it was recommended that progesterone be taken with estrogen to counteract its effects on a woman's uterus. Although natural progesterone has always been available and research regarding its benefits has been published in recognized medical literature, drug companies are not interested in a natural, non-patentable therapy like natural progesterone. Like any private enterprise, the ultimate goal of pharmaceutical companies is to make a profit - with major profits resulting largely from the sales of patented medicines. Rather than use a natural therapy, drug companies chose to formulate and promote synthetic forms of progesterone, known as progestins. Ironically, combination hormone replacement therapy (HRT) – synthetic estrogen with progestins – is now recognized as posing more of a risk to a woman's health than estrogen alone. (See Chapter 20, "Keeping Abreast of Breast Cancer.")

It is important to re-emphasize the facts outlined in Chapter Three that synthetic progestins are NEVER an appropriate substitute for endogenous progesterone (progesterone made within the body) or natural progesterone (plant-derived). The molecular structure of progestins is entirely different from progesterone and natural progesterone. Therefore, progestins are not recognized as fully compatible substances within our bodies, and for this reason often result in serious side effects. Some of progestins' side effects include cardiovascular complications, cancer, blood clots, insomnia, depression, masculinizing effects, breast tenderness, fluid retention, and edema.

Doubts Grow Regarding HRT

Despite the common perception that prescribed postmenopausal hormone replacement therapy improves the quality of life in women, the incidence of women who choose to discontinue hormone replacement therapy after the first one or two years of use is high. Recently, the *Journal of the American Medical Association* published the results of a randomized clinical study regarding postmenopausal hormone replacement therapy and quality of life. The study refuted the so-called "benefits" of prescribed hormone replacement therapy. Study participants who received hormone replacement medication had larger declines in physical function and energy compared to the placebo group. This study "should challenge the widely held belief that hormone therapy helps women remain more youthful, active, or vibrant," write Kathryn Rexrode and Jo Ann Manson of Harvard University in an accompanying editorial.[12]

Prescription forms of estrogen and progestins have been heavily promoted for everything from preventing heart attacks and osteoporosis to protecting against dementia. Yet doubts have surfaced regarding their supposed "benefits." Current research indicates that women should not expect *any* beneficial results from HRT with the exception of possibly relieving hot flashes. And if women are looking solely to eradicate hot flashes, there are safer ways of doing so.

In response to a study appearing in the June 13, 2001 volume of the *Journal of the American Medical Association* (JAMA), the USA TODAY front page headline on the same day read, "Hormone Therapy: Doubts Grow." The article highlighted that, "At the same time that HRT's benefits are becoming murkier, the potential risks are becoming more worrisome." "Why take it?" asks Dr. Stephen Cummings, M.D., co-author of an editorial accompanying the JAMA paper. "If it's for hot flashes, it's clear it works. If it's for the prevention of anything (else), it's not clear yet."[13]

Deborah Grady, M.D. and Stephen Cummings, M.D. also recently reviewed 22 studies regarding synthetic hormone replacement for osteoporosis prevention. According to their JAMA report, the validity of these studies is flawed in several important ways, rendering their results questionable. The Grady and Cummings review highlights the fact that existing evidence regarding the efficacy of postmenopausal estrogen to prevent osteoporotic fractures is tenuous. In addition, an increased incidence of cardiovascular (blood clots) and gallbladder events occurred among women on the estrogen. According to Grady and Cummings, "Since women in their fifties who do not have osteoporosis have a relatively low risk of fracture, the benefit of long-term treatment with estrogen to prevent bone loss and fractures may not exceed the risks."[14] In the end, Grady and Cummings suggest that for osteoporosis, treatments *other than* estrogen should be considered first.

The use of synthetic hormones for preventing cardiovascular events in women with or without existing heart disease has also come under fire lately. Currently, experts advise against using synthetic hormone replacement drugs with the hopes of incurring coronary benefits. Synthetic hormones have been shown to increase the development of dangerous cardiovascular events such as heart attacks, strokes, and blood clots. Due to these serious findings, in May of 2001, the National Cholesterol Education Program (NCEP) revoked their previous recommendation that synthetic hormone replacement be used for improving cholesterol status.[15] For the same reasons, the American Heart Association is no longer recommending HRT for preventing cardiovascular disease in postmenopausal women.

On a final note, the so-called evidence that prescribed hormone replacement drugs can prevent dementia and Alzheimer's disease is questionable at best. Although a number of early observational studies suggest that cognitive dysfunction or Alzheimer's disease was less prevalent in women taking postmenopausal estrogen, subsequent studies have failed to support this original theory. More recent, randomized clinical trials failed to demonstrate any benefits of estrogen for Alzheimer's disease.[16]

A Natural Solution

Scientific research, as well as anecdotal reports, reflects a dark side to traditionally prescribed hormone replacement medications. Although women continue to be plagued by menopausal symptoms, they are increasingly wary of pursuing synthetic hormones to alleviate them. With doubts increasing regarding the safety and efficacy of prescribed synthetic hormone replacement therapy, women are seeking natural options to alleviate their symptoms – effectively and without side effects.

Most North American menopausal women continue to produce reasonable levels of estrogen and may also accumulate estrogen from other sources. Yet, progesterone levels tend to hover near zero in most North American women around the time of menopause. This substantiates how many women find they are able to manage menopausal symptoms by restoring progesterone levels alone.

While there have been numerous anecdotal reports of how natural progesterone helps alleviate the symptoms of menopause, there is current scientific research regarding its value as well. Gynecologist, Dr. Ron Eaker, M.D. writes, "There is evidence that natural progesterone cream is helpful for many menopausal symptoms. Data supporting this is beginning to appear. Two papers at the recent meeting of the World Congress on Fertility and Sterility showed significant improvement in hot flashes for women using progesterone cream versus placebo. There are many anecdotal reports of its effectiveness, and I suspect that more investigations will be forthcoming."[17]

The results of a double-blind study performed by Drs. Helene Leonetti, Santo Longo, and James Anasti, published in the medical journal *Obstetrics & Gynecology*, found significant improvement in hot flash symptoms among study participants using transdermal natural progesterone.[18] In addition, a placebo-controlled double-blind study was recently conducted to determine the effect of topical progesterone cream on the endometrium (uterus lining) in postmenopausal women. Study results concluded that natural progesterone cream protected the uterus from the negative effects of estrogen and were published in a 2001 volume of the medical journal *Obstetrics & Gynecology*.[19]

The fact that natural progesterone cream exerts a distinct anti-proliferative effect on the endometrium could be of extreme value to medical experts because of the knowledge that increased cellular proliferation in any tissue of the body can raise the chances of one or more of those cells becoming cancerous. In addition, for physicians who are accustomed to prescribing progestins along with estrogen to protect the uterus from unopposed estrogen's negative effects, this study proves that natural progesterone is capable of providing protection as well, only without the numerous risk factors associated with progestin use.

For these reasons and more, natural progesterone cream is quickly becoming recognized as a viable option for women who want to safely and effectively relieve their menopausal symptoms. Researchers involved in the study regarding natural progesterone cream's anti-proliferative effects on the endometrium wrote, "Transdermal progesterone cream has become a popular alternative to [conventional] hormone replacement therapy."[20] Gynecologists like Dr. J. Ron Eaker, M.D., have already begun to use natural progesterone cream for menopausal women. Dr. Eaker states, "I have used it in my practice, specifically for hot flashes, and have seen reasonable improvement."[21] Physician and associate professor of the Obstetrical and Gynecological Department for Temple University, Dr. Helen Leonetti, M.D. states, "The most striking positive changes that I see when women start using progesterone cream are fewer mood swings, fewer hot flashes, and better sleep."[22] Being molecularly similar to the progesterone made by the body, natural progesterone offers compatibility, efficacy, and safety when used in recommended therapeutic doses.

Surely, one of the best sources of information we have regarding the beneficial effects of natural progesterone is from women themselves who have experienced them. Cheryl Roche of Wisconsin states, "I feel generally more serene. It has been helping me sleep better at night and is also helpful for my hot flashes." Again, while estrogen is still being produced in respectable levels among most menopausal women of North America, progesterone levels plunge to almost zero. Therefore, by restoring progesterone levels, classic menopausal symptoms such as hot flashes, vaginal dryness, diminished libido, and sleep disturbances are often alleviated.

I encourage women who are contemplating conventional synthetic hormone replacement to seriously consider the facts available regarding their marginal "benefits" as well as the risks involved with their use. Be reassured that synthetic hormones are not always necessary when going through menopause. Furthermore, safer, effective options exist. Above all, it is important to approach menopause holistically. Many women find that with dietary modifications, regular exercise, and supplementing with *natural* hormone therapy, they are able to achieve optimal health, wellness, and balance. (For more on natural menopause symptom management, please see Chapter 27, "The Estrogen Question.")

The Heart of the Matter: The TRUTH About HRT & Heart Disease

The impact of estrogen replacement therapy and combination hormone replacement therapy on the heart is of great concern because cardiovascular disease is the leading cause of death and a major contributor to disability in North American women.[1] Up until recently it was thought that hormone replacement drugs benefited the heart. However, pharmaceutical companies were often the source of funding for many research studies that made these claims. With their eagerness for doctors to prescribe synthetic estrogen and combination hormone replacement therapy, much of the earlier "fan-fare" was based on studies of questionable quality that may have been misrepresented.

After years of taking a supportive stance on HRT, the American Heart Association is no longer recommending that HRT be initiated for the prevention of cardiovascular disease in postmenopausal women. Nonetheless, despite the convincing, current data on this topic, synthetic hormone replacement continues to be touted as a way to prevent cardiovascular disease in postmenopausal women. "There are still a lot of people who lecture on the subject who continue to say estrogens protect against heart disease," says Dr. Isaac Schiff, *Managing Menopause* editor and head of Obstetrics and Gynecology at Boston's Massachusetts General Hospital. "I personally have never told my patients to take estrogens to prevent heart disease."[2] Lori Mosca, M.D., PhD director of preventative cardiology at New York Presbyterian Hospital in New York City and lead author of the American Heart Association science advisory states, "For many years, cardiologists and other health care providers who take care of women have assumed that HRT protects the heart. At this time, there is not sufficient evidence to make that claim."[3]

I can personally attest to the perpetuating myth that HRT helps the heart, despite strong evidence proving otherwise. I recently read through the course curriculum taught at a women's health seminar for health care professionals attended by my colleagues. Within the topic of cardiovascular disease, HRT was described as being beneficial for the heart. With health care professionals being misinformed, it is no wonder that such misinformation exists within the general public.

The Latest Research

A number of reputable studies indicating that synthetic hormone replacement does *not* prevent cardiovascular events in women with or without existing heart disease have recently been brought to the forefront. Data indicates the use of HRT drugs may actually increase the likelihood of developing heart attacks, strokes, and blood clots.

One clinical trial, the Heart and Estrogen/Progestin Replacement Study, was designed to evaluate whether hormone replacement therapy could protect postmenopausal women with heart disease from further coronary events. This randomized clinical trial followed almost 3,000 women for four years. Half were given a daily dose of estrogen and progestin while the others were assigned a placebo. After just one year, the women taking the HRT actually experienced 50 percent more heart attacks than those receiving a placebo.[4]

Clearly this study causes one to pause and question the conventional belief that estrogen alone or combination hormone replacement therapy helps prevent coronary disease in postmenopausal women. If anything, the study has proven there is more coronary risk associated with HRT usage than actual benefits. Commenting on this study, an article in an issue of the *Harvard Heart Letter* stated, "Results from the Heart Estrogen/Progestin Replacement Study turned on its ear the conventional wisdom that estrogen replacement therapy helps prevent coronary heart disease in postmenopausal women."[5]

The above study's findings, which appeared in the *Journal of the American Medical Association*, have largely discredited the original theory that synthetic hormone replacement helps prevent heart disease. Since then, doctors and researchers have eagerly awaited the results of larger, longer-term studies to help shed light on the many questions surrounding the potential risks and benefits of HRT, including whether HRT reduces the risk of cardiovascular events in women who do not have existing coronary heart disease.

The Women's Health Initiative was one of those trials experts awaited results of. More than 27,000 women between the ages of 50-79 were part of the Women's Health Initiative study. Participants were to be followed for up to eleven years with final data being made available in late 2005 or early 2006. However, on July 9, 2002, the Women's Health Initiative was abruptly ended after it became clear that HRT significantly increased the risk of breast cancer, heart disease, and strokes. Although this news sent shockwaves throughout the public and medical community, the "writing was on the wall" even three years ago.

In April of 1999, Women's Health Initiative trial investigators went to the extent of sending a letter to study participants taking synthetic hormones to alert them of their grave findings. The letter's intent was to inform participants that researchers had found a higher rate of heart attacks, strokes, and blood clots during the first two years of the study among those on HRT as compared with those in the placebo group.[6] Although unable to elaborate on details because they are not ready to be made public, Stephen Cummings, M.D. said recently, "There is going to be more from the Women's Health Initiative and it is not good."[7]

Still another current study complemented both the Heart Estrogen/Progestin Replacement Study and Women's Health Initiative findings. *The New*

England Journal of Medicine published the findings of the placebo-controlled Estrogen Replacement and Atherosclerosis Trial conducted by the Massachusetts Medical Society. This study followed about 300 women for a little over three years who were on estrogen and estrogen/progestin combination drugs. The conclusion was that neither estrogen alone nor estrogen combined with progestins prevented the progression of coronary atherosclerosis. Based on the results, researchers involved in the study advised that women should not use estrogen alone nor estrogen plus medroxyprogesterone acetate (a type of progestin known as Provera) with the expectation of any cardiovascular benefit.[8] These are compelling results to be sure. Commenting on the Estrogen Replacement and Atherosclerosis Trial, an article appearing in an issue of the *Harvard Heart Letter* stated this study "further dimmed hopes that HRT could significantly reduce heart disease risk."[9]

Finally, preliminary data from the Papworth Hormone Replacement Therapy Atherosclerosis Study, also concluded there is no cardiovascular benefit from hormone replacement therapy and possibly even a risk of increased cardiovascular events.[10] Correlating with this evidence, in her *New England Journal of Medicine* letter to the editor, Dr. Jerilynn Prior listed sixteen references disputing the claim that estrogen provided any cardiovascular benefit.[11]

Years ago, scientists discovered that estrogen increases the risk of blood clots in the legs and lungs. Since that time, inserts included in prescribed synthetic hormone medications such as the birth control pill and HRT have listed blood clots and strokes as possible side effects of taking these drugs. Dr. Jacques Rossouw, acting director of the large scale Women's Health Initiative study, attributes the increased coronary risk with estrogen replacement therapy and combination hormone replacement therapy use to estrogen's effect on blood clotting mechanisms in the body.[12] Much like in the major vessels of the legs and lungs, Rossouw suspects that estrogen also increases the probability of blood clots in the coronary vessels.

In addition to promoting blood clots, estrogen replacement therapy and combination hormone replacement therapy can also affect blood pressure. Ideally, a cell's membrane will selectively transfer potassium and magnesium into the cell while protecting against an influx of sodium. There is documentation that both estrogens and progestins can alter intracellular sodium influx and affect the renin-aldosterone system, leading to hypertension or high blood pressure. Estrogen promotes salt and water retention, thereby increasing the risk of hypertension. Hormone replacement therapy and oral contraceptives usually contain a combination of estrogen and progestins, leading to elevated plasma renin activity, subsequently raising arterial blood pressure.[13]

In contrast, progesterone not only protects against hypertension by balancing intracellular fluid, it also has an anti-stress effect on the pituitary. Progesterone is also a mild, natural diuretic and capable of improving sleep quality. In fact, after years of restless or unsettled sleep, natural progesterone's relaxing effect is one of the first benefits many women report after restoring progesterone levels. This effect can reduce stress and anxiety. In addition, natural progesterone is capable of increasing the metabolism of fats for energy by facilitating the function of the thyroid gland and has an inherent anti-inflammatory effect. Each of these actions could be beneficial to the heart.[14]

The Cholesterol Question

There is also the question of whether or not HRT may be worth taking to improve cholesterol readings. While I have seen the studies that seem to demonstrate a reduction in certain cholesterol levels with synthetic hormone use, it is important to realize that cardiovascular disease involves multiple factors and cholesterol alone has not proven to alter the progression of coronary atherosclerosis. Consider the 1995 study published in *Journal of the American Medical Association* titled, "Serum Total Cholesterol and Long-Term Coronary Heart Disease" (CHD). While estrogen does appear to lower total cholesterol, it is not clear that lowered cholesterol reduces the risk of heart disease. In addition, factors other than cholesterol play more important roles in heart disease prevention.[15]

Furthermore, while in some studies estrogen appears to decrease low-density lipoproteins ("bad" cholesterol) and increase high-density lipoproteins ("good" cholesterol), at the same time estrogen demonstrates other potentially harmful effects on the cardiovascular system. These include *increasing* triglyceride levels, *promoting* blood clots, and *raising* levels of C-reactive protein - an indicator of inflammation associated with an increased risk of cardiovascular events.[16] Clearly, cholesterol is a small piece of the heart disease puzzle. However, due largely to the effective marketing campaigns of pharmaceutical "giants," study findings regarding HRT and cholesterol have been misrepresented, giving the impression that estrogen prevents heart disease. These promotional efforts have been the impetus for widespread HRT use.

As a result of the serious findings by the recent studies showing that HRT actually increases heart attacks, strokes, and blood clots, in May of 2001 the National Cholesterol Education Program (NCEP) revoked its previous recommendation that postmenopausal women take HRT to improve cholesterol levels. The revised guideline includes "advising against the use of hormone replacement therapy." In the panel's explanation regarding this revision to their previous recommendation they write, "Studies have not shown that HRT reduces the risk for major coronary events or deaths among postmenopausal women who have heart disease. HRT also increases the risk for thromboembolism and gallbladder disease."[17]

The "Family History" Influence

Finally, I want to address the issue of women who are advised to take HRT to prevent heart disease primarily because of having a strong family history of heart disease. In many cases, women are prescribed HRT specifically to prevent heart disease because of the strong genetic links apparent in their family lines. However, the advice issued by the American Heart Association in light of recent studies is that postmenopausal women should *not* start hormone replacement therapy to protect the heart.

Those of us with medical backgrounds are familiar with "controllable" risk factors and "uncontrollable" risk factors of acquiring a particular disease. A "controllable" risk factor of a disease would be one in which a person could change (or "control") to his or her benefit or detriment. For example, one could choose to be a smoker or a nonsmoker. In the same way, one could choose to exercise or choose not to. On the other hand, an "uncontrollable" risk factor is one that is inherently "unchangeable," such as one's genetic make-up.

Years ago, when I worked on a cardiac step-down unit, I was involved with the care of cardiac patients who reportedly did "all the right things" (exercised regularly, ate "heart-healthy" diets, abstained from smoking and alcohol, etc.) in order to prevent heart disease. However, many of those patients experienced heart attacks, even necessitating open-heart surgery, due to their strong genetic history of the disease (an "uncontrollable" risk factor). This phenomenon demonstrates the challenge involved with changing or manipulating a strong genetic trait.

Therefore, it is baffling that women demonstrating a true genetic predisposition for acquiring heart disease are advised to take synthetic hormones, attaching with them the hope they will somehow afford coronary protection. The current existing data regarding the unfavorable coronary effects of prescription hormone replacement offers a slim shred of hope that it could protect the heart of a woman having a strong genetic predisposition to heart disease. Taking synthetic hormones is surely not worth the risk of developing one or more of the numerous serious side effects associated with their use as a result.

Summary

According to Rose Marie Robertson, president of the American Heart Association, the widespread use of HRT has prevented some women and physicians from relying on more important factors such as eating a heart healthy diet, exercising regularly, maintaining an appropriate body weight, and refraining from smoking in the quest to prevent heart disease.[18] It seems we would be more successful at averting the onset of coronary events or heart disease by adhering to more tried and true methods of prevention, including lifestyle changes with diet and exercise. Knowing the beneficial properties of natural progesterone, it too, may be able to offer adjunctive therapeutic coronary benefits.

Based on the latest data, it seems wise to relinquish any hope of synthetic hormone replacement medication benefiting the cardiovascular system in postmenopausal women with or without existing heart disease. On the contrary, those who choose to use synthetic hormones need to be on the alert for potentially harmful effects.

25

No Bones About It: The TRUTH About Estrogen &Osteoporosis

Many women are advised to take estrogen in order to prevent osteoporosis regardless of whether or not they experience menopausal symptoms. In fact, "osteoporosis prevention" is the main reason women over 60, who are no longer experiencing menopausal symptoms, are prescribed HRT.[1] While a deficiency of estrogen is often thought to be the main cause of osteoporosis, osteoporosis is extremely multi-factorial in origin and may develop even before the onset of menopause when estrogen levels are still normal. Furthermore, the fact that progesterone levels drop much more precipitously than estrogen at menopause is often ignored. There are numerous experts in this field who believe it has become overwhelmingly clear that the gradual decrease in levels of estrogen at menopause is *not* the cause of osteoporosis and that we have seriously misinterpreted this association.

Evidence indicates that significant bone loss can occur during the years prior to menopause (peri-menopause) - a time when estrogen levels are usually normal, yet when progesterone levels can be significantly lower. Consider the study done by endocrinologist Dr. Jerilynn Prior, M.D. that tracked pre-menopausal women for one year. Dr. Prior and her colleagues have provided reliable data demonstrating that osteoporotic bone loss frequently occurs in women with progesterone deficiency despite the presence of adequate estrogen levels. Their conclusions were that while there was no correlation between the rate of bone loss and estrogen levels, there did appear to be a link between indicators of progesterone levels and bone loss.[2] In other words, by the time a woman reaches menopause, osteoporosis can be well underway.

Many women continue to take estrogen or HRT in hopes of avoiding or delaying the onset of osteoporosis despite the fact that research studies involving the efficacy of these drugs for preventing osteoporosis have recently come under fire. In June of 2001, researchers Deborah Grady, M.D. and Stephen Cummings, M.D. from the University of California at San Fransisco, reviewed over 20 studies involving HRT and its effects on osteoporosis. Published in the *Journal of the American Medical Association*, Grady and Cummings challenged the validity of the so-called "evidence" surrounding the recommendation and use of synthetic hormone replacement for the prevention of osteoporotic fractures.

In their editorial, Grady and Cummings point out that the "evidence" is flawed by several key problems. One problem was that most of the studies were designed to test the effects of estrogen on outcomes other than bone fracture. Secondly, Grady and Cummings cited several examples explaining how many of the trials included in the meta-analysis were of questionable internal quality. Even those that were randomized, double blind studies - considered the "gold standard" of scientific research - were among those in question. Lastly, there were certain studies that simply did not involve the use of a placebo control group to afford the most accurate results.[3] Most were observational studies whereby women chose whether or not to take HRT. Observational studies are most susceptible to bias due in part to the differences between women who choose to take hormones after menopause and those who do not. Differences included access to health care, lifestyle factors, level of education, and willingness to comply with the prescribed regimen.[4]

To summarize the 22 studies' overall lack of quality, Grady and Cummings commented, "This meta-analysis highlights the fact that evidence about the efficacy of postmenopausal estrogen for prevention of osteoporotic fractures is weak. Estrogen increases the risk of venous thromboembolic events and gallbladder disease. Long-term use may increase the risk of breast cancer." They go on to state, "Until the effectiveness of estrogen is clarified, treatments other than estrogen should be the first choice for older women with osteoporosis." Their editorial concluded with the statement that, "Since women in their fifties who do not have osteoporosis have a relatively low risk of fracture, the benefit of long-term treatment with estrogen to prevent bone loss and fractures may not exceed the risks."[5]

Incidentally, while garnering less media exposure and attention than the aforementioned report, even prior to the Grady and Cummings analysis commentaries in other medical journals were already raising speculation regarding the validity of studies involving synthetic hormone use for osteoporosis prevention. In October of 2000, an article in the *Cleveland Clinic Journal of Medicine* reported that a major drawback of much of the data concerning the efficacy of estrogen for osteoporosis prevention is that it is based on case-control and cohort studies versus randomized studies which are regarded as reflecting the most valid outcomes.[6] In March of 2001, another report appearing in the *Postgraduate Medicine Journal* concurred, pointing out that an array of studies have been done to show estrogen increases bone mineral density but most of the research was obtained from less accurate retrospective, case-control studies in which fracture sites were often combined to arrive at the total fracture risk. In addition, the article indicated that dosages and length of therapy were extremely variable, making the comparison and conclusion of results difficult.[7]

To further demonstrate the lack of evidence supporting the use of HRT for osteoporosis prevention, the *American Journal of Medicine* recently published the results of a study entitled, "Effects of Hormone Replacement Therapy on Clinical Fractures and Height Loss." Unlike most of the other studies, this study was a large, randomized trial – the type known for producing the most accurate data. The conclusion was that after four years of treatment, hormone replacement therapy did not reduce the incidence of fractures or prevent height loss.[8] Dr. Jacques Rossouw, lead project director of the Women's Health Initiative agrees. "If one of my women friends asks me 'what should I do for osteoporosis?' I don't advise estrogen."[9]

Nutritional Role in Osteoporosis Prevention

Nutrition is an important factor to consider in osteoporosis prevention. Nutrients such as calcium, magnesium, zinc, phosphorus, and vitamins D, C, and A play important roles in the dietary prevention of osteoporosis. Calcium, in particular, plays a significant role because of its bone-building action. However, just like with estrogen, there are misconceptions about the part calcium plays in the prevention of osteoporosis.

Because it is now recognized that osteoporosis prevention needs to take place early in life, more consumer products are being targeted specifically to convince young women the products will help delay or even prevent the onset of osteoporosis. However, contrary to popular belief, osteoporosis may be due more to calcium *loss* than to actual calcium deficiency.[10] This means that despite how much calcium one consumes, certain factors can inhibit calcium's effectiveness. Persons who smoke, have diets high in protein (the excretion of protein waste products via the kidneys increases the urinary excretion of calcium, also known as "negative calcium balance"), or who take drugs that promote the loss of calcium or inhibit its absorption, may not be able to maintain adequate calcium levels to keep bones strong and healthy.

It is also critically important to obtain calcium through quality sources that include magnesium. Calcium must be absorbed into the bones to do its intended job and, unbeknownst to many, magnesium plays a crucial role in osteoporosis prevention due to its action of facilitating calcium into the bone. While compiling research for this book, I came across medical experts who consider a lack of *magnesium* to play more of a role in the development of osteoporosis than a lack of calcium. Although there are many foods, drinks, and vitamin supplements that boast "high calcium content," the truth is that these products usually lack the essential amounts of magnesium to make the calcium work effectively. Therefore, even though a product may contain high amounts of calcium, the question becomes whether or not it also contains sufficient amounts of magnesium to actually direct the calcium into the bone to promote optimum bone health.

Probably the most prevalent example of the myth that "calcium alone is enough," is the claim made by advertisements that the calcium contained in certain chewable antacids "builds bones" and "prevents osteoporosis." Promoting these products as quality sources of calcium is a well-known advertising strategy known as *positioning*. In reality, chewable antacids are among some of the poorest sources of calcium available. They do not contain adequate amounts of magnesium to facilitate calcium absorption into the bone. Although the health care industry should know better, this advertising ploy has obviously been extremely effective for the product manufacturers involved. It is surprising how many women tell me they have been advised to take TUMS specifically to promote bone health!

Furthermore, antacids can negatively affect calcium levels by inhibiting the body's ability to absorb calcium and other important nutrients. In order for calcium and other nutrients to be properly absorbed, adequate amounts of stomach acid are necessary. It is a fact that digestive juices, including hydrochloric acid found in the stomach, are utilized to help break down and absorb food into our body systems. Because antacids block or suppress the secretion of stomach acid, they may actually inhibit adequate absorption of vitamins and nutrients vital to optimum functioning. In addition, contrary to what the makers of chewable antacids and the oral forms of H2 blockers would have us think, it is incorrect to suggest that stomach acid is the primary cause of indigestion and ulcers. A lack of hydrochloric acid in the stomach can impair the digestion process and bacteria have been implicated in causing ulcers.

A final point regarding calcium has to do with the refined sugar found in many of the products marketed specifically for their high calcium content. The concept of obtaining calcium via sugary drinks and foods may seem appealing at first, but is deceiving. The considerable amounts of refined sugar found in many of these products often do more harm than good based upon the low levels of calcium they contain. Studies demonstrate how refined sugar can actually deplete calcium stores, making the potential benefits of calcium virtually counteracted by the sugar in some products.[11]

Finally, vitamin D is another important factor in building strong, healthy bones. Vitamin D interacts with calcium and phosphorus to facilitate bone mineralization, an important step in the bone-building process. Sunlight is one of the best sources of vitamin D because it facilitates the process of vitamin D production. Just a few minutes of sun exposure each day will often be enough to supply the body with adequate doses of this essential vitamin.

The "Family History" Factor

Another topic I want to address is the issue of women who take synthetic hormone replacement because of a strong family history of osteoporosis. First of all, it is questionable whether estrogen even plays a role in osteoporosis prevention based on the latest research findings. Secondly, if there truly exists a strong genetic predisposition to developing osteoporosis, and not simply a family trait of poor dietary or exercise habits, it would seem unlikely that simply supplementing with estrogen could afford a woman the assurance of averting the onset of this disease - surely not without the threat of developing side effects from its use. Furthermore, to most women, the risk of developing osteoporosis is a less frightening prospect than the risk of being stricken with cancer. Although osteoporosis can be a potentially debilitating disease, it is certainly not inherently deadly.

Weighing the Risks vs. "Benefits"

I strongly encourage any woman trying to make an educated decision about whether or not to take HRT for osteoporosis prevention to closely examine the lack of conclusive evidence regarding its value for this purpose as well as the serious side effects and risk factors that commonly occur with prescribed HRT use. Clearly, there are other factors that have been identified over the years that play more of a significant role in the prevention of osteoporosis including nutrition, weight bearing exercise, and progesterone levels.

What many fail to recognize is that progesterone, which levels drop much more significantly at menopause than estrogen, may actively increase bone mass and density. Dr. John Lee, M.D. explains, "in late 1979, I began recommending progesterone cream to my osteoporotic patients who could not use estrogen. Using annual serial dual photon bone absorptiometry (DPA) tests, I followed the bone condition of these patients. To my considerable surprise, the bone mineral density tests showed that my patients using progesterone cream showed significant increase (average 15%) whereas my patients on estrogen alone showed no increase but either remained stable or actually decreased." The following letter published in a current issue of the John R. Lee, M.D. Medical Letter testifies to what he has observed in his practice.

Two years ago my mother was diagnosed with severe osteoporosis. She was 74 years old and had lost about two inches in height. Her doctor immediately wanted to start her on Fosamax. Instead, I suggested (after having read all your books and following your suggestion for PMS, which has been miraculous for me) natural progesterone cream. We increased her intake of a mineral supplement, and she continued her three-mile walks per day. My mother just got back the results of her bone density test today and her new doctor said she never saw such an improvement! Her left femoral went from −3.09 to −2.1 and her L2 and L4 region went from -.43 to +0.6. Mom is 76 years old and is doing great…[12]

Summary – "The Bigger Picture"

Clearly, osteoporosis is a multi-factorial disease that can be prevented in many cases. According to the most current literature and research, it seems that restoring progesterone, along with a conscientious diet (one in which the dietary factors influencing osteoporosis are considered), a quality nutritional supplement, and regular weight-bearing exercise could safely support the maintenance of bone mass as well as promote new bone formation. These factors would likely contribute to the prevention and possibly even the reversal of osteoporosis.

Without a doubt, there is something mistaken about the "estrogen theory." The "evidence" of estrogen's benefits in preventing osteoporosis is not convincing. In addition, estrogen use may increase the risk of cancer, blood clots, cardiac abnormalities, headaches, weight gain, gallbladder disease, and other health concerns. Therefore, it would seem unlikely that women should ever truly need to take estrogen or HRT solely for the prevention of osteoporosis. Furthermore, it is never prudent to rely on a single method for disease prevention. One must consider the "bigger picture," lest we forget that osteoporosis involves multiple factors. It is up to you to educate yourself on the significance each factor plays and develop an individualized plan of protection against this potentially debilitating disease.

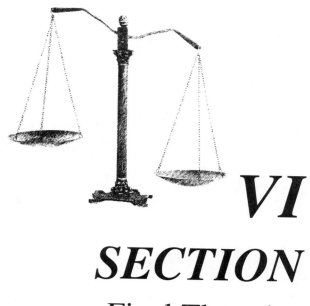

VI
SECTION
Final Thoughts

26

The Problem with "the Pill" & other Chemical Contraceptives

At one point in time, I ended up taking the birth control pill (which I will refer to as simply "the pill") for about a month. I remember it clearly because it was the month after I became married. Like millions of other women, I easily obtained a prescription from my family physician who explained that it was a convenient and effective form of birth control. Yet, having a friend who experienced a blood clot as a result of taking the pill, I expressed concern about potential side effects and questioned my doctor about them. I was told that side effects were rare and, based on my health history, I had very little to be concerned about. That was all I needed to hear. Off I went to the local drug store to fill my prescription for what was considered to be a "low-dose" oral contraceptive.

I took my prescription faithfully and found that it was fairly convenient, while at the same time affording adequate protection against pregnancy. However, to my surprise and dismay, the entire time I took the pill I did not feel like my "normal" self at all. I was unusually fatigued, crabby, and experienced vaginal dryness as well as a lack of libido. Referring to the small piece of paper that accompanied my prescription, I discovered my symptoms listed among the many potential side effects.

Returning to the doctor, I explained my experience and discussed alternative birth control options – none of which would involve drugs. I cannot tell you how relieved I was to return to feeling "normal" again the following month. Although I didn't know as much then as I know now about the pill, I discovered first-handedly the way in which it distorts our body's natural design enough to never want to be on it again.

Strong Hormones, Strong Effects

Think about the fact that our bodies naturally produce significant levels of incredibly strong hormones in order to have the capability of creating and sustaining a living, breathing, human being. Because of this, in order to prevent ovulation from occurring, a much stronger dose of hormones is required. This stronger dose of hormones is achieved with the use of chemical contraceptives like the birth control pill. With chemical contraceptives, the intricate processes of the reproductive organs become completely dictated by powerful, synthetic hormones. It is difficult to fully comprehend the quantity of potent, synthetic hormones that are delivered on a consistent basis, suppressing the body's ability to ovulate and sustain a human life. I have heard one women's health expert describe the birth control pill's mechanism of action as the "chemical castration" of females.

My goal is to convey to women the sheer magnitude of powerful, synthetic hormones that are found in birth control pills yet I frequently encounter replies of, "I happen to be on the 'lowest dosage' available." I respond by explaining that even in the lowest dosages available, birth control pills still contain very potent levels of unnatural, synthetic hormones making them powerful enough to literally overtake your body's own hormones, thereby sending the ovaries into an anovulatory state.

By using birth control pills or other forms of chemical contraceptives, a woman's body drastically deviates from the way it was designed to function. When under the influence of birth control pills, the state of a young woman's body can be likened to a type of "menopause." Yet even during menopause, the ovaries are still producing hormones. With the pill, the ovaries' ability to produce hormones is arrested. In other words, by taking the pill, a steady dose of powerful, synthetic hormones, usually in the form of synthetic estrogen and progestins combined, are delivered to your body on a daily basis, literally shutting down all sex hormone production. At the same time there is a risk for developing a host of dangerous or even life threatening side effects.

Contraceptive injections and implants, such as Depo-Provera and Norplant, take this concept a step further. These injections and implants deliver such enormous doses of synthetic hormones that one's own hormones are overcome and virtually shut down for several months or years at a time. The strength of synthetic hormones found in these drugs defies comprehension. As with the pill, women who are given contraceptive injections or implants risk developing unfavorable effects. The teenage daughter, of a woman at one of my seminars, was given the Depo-Provera injection to "treat" her severe menstrual cramps. As a result, the girl ended up bleeding the entire three months she was on it. The college-aged daughter of another woman I met at a recent lecture of mine explained that she, too, has bled non-stop since receiving the Depo injection.

Chemical Contraceptives' Link to Infertility

Unfortunately, one of the most disheartening side effects of using chemical contraceptives can be infertility. *"The Couple's Guide to Fertility"* by Gary S. Berger, M.D. states, "Long-term pill users may not menstruate or ovulate after they stop using the pill. This condition, known as *post-pill amenorrhea* occurs because the pill disrupts the natural rhythmic flow of hormones from the hypothalamus to the pituitary to the ovaries. This may pose a special problem for women who have been on the pill for many years because their ovaries may have become resistant to resuming ovulation."[1]

The human body is "smart," abiding by the "use it or lose it" rule of thumb. If the sex hormones produced by the ovaries are suppressed for a long enough period - a time frame that can vary from woman to woman - the body interprets this to mean that they are no longer needed and the ovaries may eventually stop functioning. As mentioned earlier, Fabio

Bertarelli, owner of Serano Labs which manufacture 70 percent of the world's fertility drugs, told the *Wall Street Journal* in 1993, "Our usual customers are women over 30 who have been taking birth control pills since they were teenagers or in their early twenties."[2] How sad but true this is. I cannot help but think that if these women had been made aware of these facts beforehand, most would have elected not to take the pill - at least not for so long.

Additional Concerns

In addition to fertility concerns, other side effects that occur with the use of chemical contraceptives can be found in any PDR *(Physicians Desk Reference)*. These side effects include, but are not limited to, blood clots which can lead to a stroke, heart attacks, headaches and migraines, high blood pressure, cancer (breast, cervical, endometrial), altered immune function, abdominal pain and tenderness, gallbladder disease, and decreased glucose tolerance. Depression is another condition known to occur with chemical contraceptive use because the progestins, frequently combined with estrogen in these drugs, can interfere with serotonin production. A deficiency of serotonin has been found to coincide with depression.[3] Oral contraceptives and Depo-Provera injections have also been implicated in increasing the risk of women developing certain vaginal infections such as chlamydia or yeast.[4]

Of particular concern is how chemical contraceptive use can affect nutrient levels within the body. Those who take synthetic hormonal contraceptives tend to have lower levels of vitamin B6, folic acid, vitamin B12, vitamin B2, and beta-carotene, an important antioxidant.[5] Deficiencies in magnesium and manganese can also occur from the synthetic estrogen supplied by these drugs. This phenomenon can contribute to the development of headaches and migraines and is discussed in more detail in Chapter Six.

I gave the example in Chapter Seven of a 23 year-old woman named Rose who began taking the pill after getting married. Rose soon developed headaches, gained a significant amount of weight, and experienced depression. The synthetic hormones found in the birth control pill are known to cause all of the symptoms Rose experienced. Yet, Rose was prescribed three additional medications in an effort to eliminate her symptoms. Her prescriptions included a migraine headache medication (an injection), a thyroid replacement medication (Synthroid), and an antidepressant (Prozac). Quite likely, if Rose's body had never been subject to the strong doses of synthetic hormones from the birth control pill, she may have been able to avoid her subsequent health problems, as well as the additional medications.

Lastly, but certainly not least, cancer is associated with the synthetic hormones found in the pill and other chemical contraceptives. The association between oral contraceptives and the risk of breast cancer has been studied extensively. Drs. Mark Clemons and Paul Goss wrote a comprehensive report explaining the relationship between prescription hormones and breast cancer in a recent volume of the *New England Journal of Medicine*. In their report they point out that four current double-blind studies have demonstrated an association to breast cancer either overall or in subgroups of women who have taken oral contraceptives for a long time, as well as those who started taking oral contraceptives at an early age.[6]

Another study, reported on in the *Journal of the American Medical Association*, found that users of the birth control pill were three times more likely than nonusers to get breast cancer if there was a strong family history of the disease.[7] In other words, the pill raises the already heightened risk of breast cancer in women with a strong genetic link to the disease.

Finally, a current volume of *Gynecological Endocrinology* published a study revealing a 30 percent increase in women developing cervical dysplasia with oral contraceptive use. Abnormal cervical cells are considered precursers to cervical cancer.

Cancer seems to be the most feared of all diseases in North America – and with good reason. As mortality rates climb, it is clear that we are not winning this battle with current conventional treatment modalities. To reduce cancer incidence and mortality rates, we need to focus on prevention. In particular, it would be helpful if specific information was widely disseminated regarding known carcinogens such as the synthetic hormones found in chemical contraceptives. These drugs have powerful effects on the body, yet with education and increased awareness, many could be avoided.

"Closing Arguments"

We have become a society that thrives on the "quick fix" for anything from a broken down vehicle to our own health. No longer is the use of birth control pills and other chemical contraceptives reserved solely for preventing pregnancies. Instead, they are commonly prescribed for "treating" a variety of conditions and symptoms. These include hormone-related problems such as certain types of acne, endometriosis, ovarian cysts, uterine fibroids, heavy periods, menstrual cramps, and irregular bleeding - conditions that are often resolved by restoring hormone balance.

There is no question that birth control pills and other chemical contraceptives act quickly. These drugs are often effective in the short run because of how they immediately shut down ovarian hormone production. For example, if a woman is experiencing heavy menstrual bleeding or painful menstrual cramping, chemical contraceptives will abruptly halt the onset of her natural menstrual cycle, thus eliminating the chance for symptoms to persist. In the long run, however, chemical contraceptives place women at risk for experiencing one or more of the numerous serious side effects associated with their use.

Although it may take time to form a definitive diagnosis or determine a likely underlying reason for the onset of a particular symptom, doing so is superior to simply eliminating the symptom as a "quick fix." In many cases, symptoms can serve as a "warning system" and by heeding the body's "warning," we are able to take affirmative action in curing the problem. In other words, correcting the underlying causes of health concerns versus simply eliminating symptoms (symptom-based treatment) avoids the possibility of "masking" serious health problems. In addition, once the origin of symptoms and conditions is discovered, future prevention becomes a possibility.

While it may be difficult to find a birth control method that is both as effective and convenient as chemical contraceptives are, I still encourage couples to consider other options. I consistently maintain that the advantages of chemical contraceptives come with a potential price to pay. The price to pay may range from mildly annoying symptoms such as mood swings, headaches, and vaginal dryness, to life-changing conditions like infertility, to life-threatening health problems including weight gain, blood clots, and cancer. The choice is ultimately yours. The choice involves weighing what you value most in life and what you are willing to sacrifice as a result.

TWENTY SEVEN 27

The Estrogen Question

Because so much of what I have covered in this book involves reasons why it may be worth avoiding most forms of estrogen, I fear being accused of suggesting that no one should ever take estrogen. Therefore, I want to set the record straight regarding what literature indicates to satisfactorily answer the question, "Is there ever a good reason for a woman to supplement with estrogen?"

Examining Estrogen Levels

Several years ago, a study by Dr. Stephen Cummings at Harvard indicated that two-thirds of postmenopausal women continue to make sufficient amounts of estrogen up to the age of 80. In other words, only about one-third of postmenopausal women are considered truly "estrogen-deficient."[1] Dr. Helene Leonetti, M.D., a private practice physician and associate professor of obstetrics and gynecology at Temple University, has discovered similar findings in her clinical practice. In regards to her past nine years of practice she says, "I'd estimate that I've put over 12,000 patients on [natural] progesterone, and they almost universally adore it. Between 25 and 35 percent of my patients are on estrogen and progesterone. The rest are on progesterone alone because most of them are estrogen dominant. Women who continue with hot flashes and other symptoms of estrogen deficiency who just don't feel balanced, I put on estrogen."[2]

Estradiol, Estrone, and Estriol

Not all estrogens act precisely the same in our bodies. Among the three major estrogens, *estradiol* and *estrone* are recognized as the most carcinogenic, while *estriol* is recognized as the least carcinogenic. In

1996, a study published in the *Journal of the American Medical Association* described estriol as having more benign effects compared to more harmful estrogens like estrone and estradiol, commonly prescribed under the names Premarin, Estraderm, and Esterace.[3] Another medical journal recently reported that estriol is the "weakest" estrogen found in the body and may prove to provide protection against breast cancer.[4] During pregnancy, estriol and progesterone are the predominant hormones produced. It is ironic that the two hormones that predominate during the course of a woman's pregnancy are shown to be protective against cancer, yet they are the same two hormones least likely to be recommended for the treatment of menopausal symptoms in lieu of the more harmful synthetic counterparts! Clearly, estriol and progesterone are respectable options when considering hormone replacement.

Phytoestrogens

The chemical classification for phytoestrogens is a misnomer because they lack a steroidal nucleus found in estrogen. Unbeknownst to many, phytoestrogens are not estrogens at all, nor are they converted to estrogen by the body. On the contrary, phytoestrogens are compounds manufactured by various plants that can have hormonal effects. They are primarily comprised of the class of compounds known as isoflavones and flavones.[5] Isoflavones and flavones have been found to interact with estrogen receptors, demonstrating weak yet beneficial estrogenic effects. Isoflavones, such as soy, act to displace stronger and more toxic estrogens in breast cell receptor sites. Soy also contains *protease inhibitors* that may slow cancer division rates and *saponins* that may prevent cancer cell multiplication.

Scientific research involving phytoestrogens can be difficult to interpret due to a number of confounding factors. Although these factors make some aspects of phytoestrogens the subject of debate, there is research that indicates phytoestrogens can be beneficial. Research demonstrates how phytoestrogens often act like a weak form of estrogen, competing for and occupying estrogen receptors, even offering the possibility of protection against cancer. There is epidemiological evidence that because Asian women consume traditional diets high in soy, they experience fewer menopausal symptoms as well as a much lower incidence of breast cancer than European or Western women. Phytoestrogens have been implicated in reducing hot flashes, vaginal dryness, and the incidence of breast cancer. They may also help to alleviate other symptoms of menopause including sleep difficulties and mood disorders.

In some respects, phytoestrogens seem to replicate the actions of SERMs (selective estrogen receptor modulators) – a class of drugs said to mimic some of estrogen's beneficial effects (like alleviating symptoms of hot flashes) while perhaps preventing cancer. Because estrogens and estrogenic substances all compete for the same receptor sites within the body, it is possible that this phenomenon - phytoestrogens' ability to occupy estrogen receptor sites - could protect against more harmful estrogens that would otherwise occupy the same receptor sites. In other words, if estrogen receptor sites are occupied by the "weaker" or more "benign" estrogenic agents, the carcinogenic effects of estrogens like estrone and estradiol, or those that stem from the environment in the form of toxic estrogenic compounds, may be derailed.

Because of their beneficial properties, phytoestrogens may be worth considering as an alternative to traditional hormone replacement therapy when seeking to restore estrogen levels. The idea of feeding a tumor seems to be the single most common reason women are reluctant to begin a regimen of prescription estrogen replacement therapy. Increasing dietary phytoestrogen intake or incorporating a natural phytoestrogen supplement may be beneficial options. It is becoming increasingly common to hear of women controlling their menopausal symptoms by altering their diets -

incorporating more soy, fresh fruits and vegetables, as well as whole grains. In addition, there are women who prefer to use a natural phytoestrogen supplement specifically formulated for use during menopause. These supplements can be in the form of tablets or creams and may be used alone or in combination with natural progesterone to ward off menopausal symptoms

Factors of Maintaining and Supplementing Estrogen Levels

It is important to recognize other ways estrogen levels are maintained in the body without necessarily supplementing with prescription estrogen medication. In addition to the ovaries, a woman's body secretes or stores estrogen in the adrenal glands, fat cells, and liver throughout her lifetime. On the contrary, the only ongoing postmenopausal source of progesterone is the adrenal glands. Yet a stressful lifestyle can challenge the adrenals' ability to produce sufficient amounts of progesterone.

It is also true that when a woman supplements with natural progesterone, the presence of progesterone makes certain body tissues more sensitive to estrogen. As a result, the "need" for supplemental estrogen may no longer exist.[6] In other words, once progesterone levels are raised, estrogen receptors often become more sensitive, and menopausal symptoms like hot flashes and vaginal dryness can be alleviated. Therefore, once progesterone is added, many postmenopausal women, with or without ovaries, do not require estrogen supplementation.

Certainly if symptoms or the results of a saliva hormone assay indicate a probable estrogen deficiency, it may be appropriate to consider estrogen supplementation with discretion. Ideally, estrogen supplementation would take place using one of the agents considered least carcinogenic, in the lowest dosage to obtain the desired effect, and always in combination with *natural* progesterone (not progestins) versus being "unopposed" (estrogen taken alone or without progesterone). Recall the statement made by the Mayo Clinic in the 1970s regarding how unopposed estrogen replacement therapy increases the risk of cancer. Also, in regards to unopposed estrogen, Dr. David Zava, Ph.D., a highly respected breast cancer researcher for over 30 years, has stated,

> Unopposed estrogen therapy is truly iatrogenic [doctor-induced] illness at its worst. In most cases the entire domino effect,

from estrogen dominance to overgrowth of the endometrial lining, to hysterectomy, to severe hormonal imbalance and estrogen dominance caused by supplementation with unopposed estrogens, to excessive and unnecessary medications for depression and anxiety, to bone loss, could have been avoided if these women had known to use progesterone from the beginning.[7]

Considering the latest data and clinical evidence, it seems wise to avoid prescribed synthetic hormones when possible. Women should know that they can effectively relieve menopausal symptoms and prevent the onset of conditions like osteoporosis and heart disease through safer methods (diet, exercise, natural progesterone, etc.). It is also important to remember that the ovaries do not entirely stop producing estrogen at menopause nor do they "die and wither away." In most cases, the ovaries continue to make respectable amounts of estrogen (and testosterone), just not enough to initiate the menstrual cycle. While there are women with an estrogen deficiency, supplemental estrogen in a woman who does not need it or who is not balancing it with natural sources of progesterone can lead to a number of estrogen dominant symptoms including water retention, fibrocystic breasts, headaches, depression, weight gain, gallbladder problems, and hormone related cancers.[8]

Knowing that estrogen levels can be maintained in a variety of ways, the only question that remains is - is it enough estrogen? Once again, if clinical symptoms persist or a saliva hormone assay indicates an estrogen deficiency relative to progesterone, it may be beneficial to supplement with estrogen. In these cases, it is recommended to use an estrogen known to have the least carcinogenic effects, in the lowest dosage to achieve results, and never unopposed, but rather in combination with *natural* progesterone.

Be patient as well as creative when attempting to determine the appropriate amount of estrogen your body requires. Instead of taking an estrogen pill or using an estrogen patch every day, it may be helpful to experiment with an every other day schedule. One woman I know has achieved balance by using her estrogen patch for just several hours each day in conjunction with a natural progesterone therapy regimen. It is important to keep in mind that every body is uniquely designed with unique needs!

Summary

28

Why a Cream?

I cannot end this book without addressing the purpose of using a natural progesterone cream versus other forms of natural progesterone. I am often asked, "Why a cream? Why not just take a pill?"

It is important to realize that the skin is the largest organ of the human body. On its surface are millions of tiny pores that act much like absorbent sponges. Below the skin's surface you will find a vast supply of blood. Anything that is applied onto the skin's outer surface is capable of being absorbed into the innermost layers and then efficiently transported throughout the entire body via the remarkable circulatory system. That is why we need to pay particular attention to what we apply onto our skin (such as makeup, lotions, soaps, and medications), just as we do to what we put into our mouths.

While it is true that under the right circumstances, the skin is an effective "transportation system" for medications and other therapies, absorption rates can vary among persons as well as among body sites. For example, if a person routinely applies body lotions or "moisturizers" containing mineral oil or other petroleum derivatives, they are actually applying a barrier or "film" onto the skin's surface that will prevent penetration of any other substance into the pores (this is why moisturizers containing mineral oil or petrolatum do not effectively moisturize). Knowing this, it would be very difficult or even impossible for a natural progesterone cream to be properly absorbed under these circumstances.

Therefore, it is best to avoid using products containing petroleum derivatives especially while using natural progesterone cream because of how they can interfere with the absorption process. More importantly, petroleum derivative products are among the growing list of substances considered to be *estrogenic compounds* – substances that occupy the estrogen receptors in our bodies, leading to potentially harmful estrogen excess effects.

One of the primary reasons cream-based therapies have been a target of criticism is due to the claim that they are not well absorbed transdermally. However, it is interesting that for years drugs have been administered in a cream base (such as Nitropaste) as well as in the form of transdermal patches for smoking cessation, depression, and hormone replacement. There is also sound scientific research that demonstrates how hormones like progesterone are effectively absorbed transdermally (see Chapter 20, "Keeping Abreast of Breast Cancer"). Recently, I even learned about a synthetic estrogen and progestin patch intended for use as a form of birth control by Johnson & Johnson. Research shows it is absorbed well enough through the skin to be a reliable form of contraception!

Clearly, we are seeing an increasing number of prescription drugs in the forms of creams and transdermal patches because of the convenience and effectiveness they afford in delivering the drug where it needs to go. Being fat-soluble, natural progesterone is particularly well absorbed through the skin, especially in "soft tissue" areas. These areas include the face, neck, chest, breasts, inner arms, inner thighs, palms of the hands, and the insoles of the feet.

Conversely, because progesterone is fat-soluble, when administered orally, it is taken up by the portal vein and transported directly to the liver where up to 80 to 90 percent of it can be lost.[1] As a result, oral forms of progesterone must often be taken in higher dosages (usually 100mg – 200mg per day) than when administered transdermally (20mg - 40mg per day) in order to be comparatively effective in achieving normal physiologic levels. The higher doses required with oral forms of progesterone subsequently place a greater workload upon the liver.[2] I recently spoke to a registered pharmacist who confirmed that natural progesterone has a much higher level of bioavailability when administered transdermally instead of orally. In other words, the body is able to utilize progesterone much more efficiently when it is administered in the form of a transdermal cream rather than via a pill.

TWENTY NINE

29

The "Bigger Picture": Other Factors for Optimal Health

Although the focus of my research involves hormone balance, the reader should understand that I fully recognize and appreciate the integral roles other factors like nutrition and exercise play in achieving optimal health. In addition to the benefits of maintaining hormone balance, it is wise to consider the value of a healthy diet and regular exercise when seeking to stay on the path of wellness.

Growing up in a home where my mother was fiercely committed to putting only the purest foods into our bodies, I have always been keenly aware of the significance in the motto, "we are what we eat." With that in mind, I realize that phrases like, "a healthy diet" and "good nutrition" mean different things to different people. These phrases can define anything from eating the correct number of servings from each food group on a daily basis, to eating only those foods which are considered "low fat and low cholesterol," to eating strictly vegetarian or organic. Surely, if I were to ask ten different people what they felt was meant by the phrase "a healthy diet" I would receive ten different responses.

Certain diets have been found to be protective against cancer. Generally speaking, diets high in fiber, fruits, and vegetables have been found to protect against cancer. In addition, cultures with low cancer rates usually obtain 20 percent or less of their daily calorie intake from fat. Phytoestrogens are also a dietary mainstay of people in these cultures. Soy contains *isoflavones*, phytoestrogens that displace stronger and more toxic estrogens in breast cell receptor sites. Soy also contains *protease inhibitors* and *saponins* that may prevent cancer cells from multiplying and growing. Flaxseeds contain lignans that are converted into phytoestrogens, which also may offer cancer protection by blocking more powerful estrogens in the body.[1]

Obviously, there is much I could say about nutrition and diet. To me a healthy diet means plenty of fresh fruits and vegetables as well as whole grains, eaten as unprocessed as possible and uncontaminated by pesticides, refined sugar, artificial coloring, flavoring agents, or preservatives. Consuming plenty of pure, fresh water is also very important. In addition, I am convinced that most people can benefit from a quality nutritional supplement on a daily basis. Even if you consider your diet to be generally healthy, taking a quality nutritional supplement simply affords an added measure of protection against nutritional deficiencies, environmental toxins, and the stresses of everyday life.

Exercise

I once heard a prominent female obstetrician gynecologist state that the key to "staying young" was to exercise regularly. Clearly, exercise is a great way to improve health and wellness. Not only does it build strong bones and tone muscles (including the heart muscle), as well as increase energy and stamina, regular exercise relieves stress and promotes healthy cells by delivering generous doses of oxygen and nutrients via the circulatory system. Exercise has even proven to boost immunity and resistance against infection. Furthermore, exercise can decrease body fat. Excess body fat can be a source of excess estrogen because estrogen is stored in fat cells. Therefore, the loss of body fat can contribute to decreased estrogen levels and a healthier balance of hormones.

As with the phrase "healthy diet," "regular exercise" can mean different things to different people. In the preoperative teaching program where I currently work, one of the questions I am required to ask patients planning an upcoming surgery is, "Do you engage in a regular exercise program?" While some folks answer with a simple "yes" or "no," others go on to describe what their exercise regimen entails. Many young mothers feel that "chasing around the kids all day" constitutes of regular exercise, just as those who work in a store or restaurant perceive that "being on my feet all day" is enough exercise.

Most of the literature on exercise seems to identify the ideal exercise program as consisting of a combination of cardiovascular (aerobic), strength training (weights), and stretching exercises three or four times a week. While some of us cannot fathom the idea of exercising that often, even a small amount of regular exercise is better than none at all.

Summary

Our hormones are constantly fluctuating due to intrinsic and extrinsic factors, affecting our lives and health in numerous ways. However, hormone balance is only one piece of the puzzle. There can exist a false sense of security when a person puts his or her faith in a single factor to promote wellness as well as to prevent or treat disease. Let us never overlook the "bigger picture." Clearly, it is prudent to consider the important roles factors such as nutrition and exercise play when planning an individualized plan of action to achieve and maintain optimal health and wellness throughout our lifetimes.

Conclusion

I encourage you to use the information I have provided to consider the possibility of hormones and/or hormone imbalance being involved in the predominant health concerns facing women today. In addition, I challenge you to consider the benefits in preventing, diagnosing, and treating the underlying etiologies of these symptoms and conditions by taking steps to restore hormone balance safely and naturally. Above all, listen to what your body is "telling" you and strive for a body functioning in balance and harmony.

Keep in mind that while much progress has been made in understanding the concepts of hormone imbalance, there remains more to discover and understand. It is important to stay educated. While I don't claim to have all the answers, I hope to have given you an introduction to the facts available today.

Thank you for your interest in the topic of hormone balance. I welcome your comments. Feel free to visit my website at www.lifeandhealth.myarbonne.com. To obtain additional copies of this book, call 1-800-964-8865 and request item #GB030.

Kristine Klitzke, RN, BSN

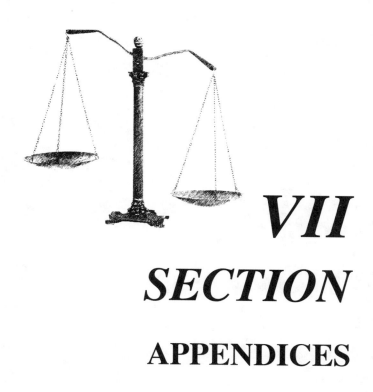

VII

SECTION

APPENDICES

APPENDIX A

Just the Facts: Quick Answers to Commonly Asked Questions

While answers to the following questions are explained in more detail throughout the book, I have included this format to be utilized as a quick reference. For "the rest of the story," I strongly encourage you to read the entire book or refer to specific chapters.

Q What exactly is meant by the term "estrogen dominance" and why should it be assessed for?

Estrogen dominance describes a condition of hormone imbalance whereby the normal ratios of estrogen and progesterone are altered due to excess estrogen and/or inadequate progesterone. Studies done by the World Health Organization have indicated that women in Westernized cultures like North America tend to have high levels of estrogen relative to progesterone due to a variety of exogenous and endogenous factors (described in Chapter Four). Because there is current, reputable data clearly demonstrating that excess estrogen and/or a progesterone deficiency can exert detrimental effects on the body in a variety of ways, an underlying condition of estrogen dominance should be routinely assessed for.

Q What are the symptoms and/or conditions that can occur as a result of estrogen dominance?

Symptoms and conditions of estrogen dominance can include but are not limited to PMS, water retention, breast swelling, breast tenderness, fibrocystic breasts, irritability, mood swings, depression, loss of libido, heavy or irregular menses, uterine fibroids, cervical dysplasia, fatigue, headaches, and unexplained weight gain. Conditions such as fibromyalgia, chronic fatigue, thyroid disorders, and autoimmune diseases are also closely associated with estrogen dominance. In addition, estrogen dominance is known to be a factor in many types of cancer such as breast, uterine (endometrial), cervical, ovarian, and prostate.

Q How can one know with some certainty that a specific symptom and/or condition is due to estrogen dominance and not to something else?

Hormones made by the body are bound by protein so they can be carried in the blood. These protein-bound hormones are not entirely biologically active. The more revelant component is the 1-10 percent of "unbound" hormone which is biologically active and present in saliva. Also, when absorbed transdermally, progesterone is not coated with this protein. Thus, while transdermal progesterone levels may not be readily detected in a serum (blood) test, they are quickly detected in saliva. Therefore, given the option of saliva hormone testing versus assessing hormone levels via a blood test – a saliva reading would provide a more accurate measurement. Saliva hormone assays can often provide more relevant data than serum tests for assessing hormone levels.

Whether blood or saliva hormone assays are performed, because each of us is unique in body frame, metabolism rates, etc., it is uncertain if a "normal" level for me would also be a "normal" level for someone else. In addition, saliva hormone tests are quite specific and are helpful only when analyzed correctly. They measure only true estrogens, endogenous progesterone, and progesterone that is bio-identical to endogenous progesterone (USP natural progesterone). Hormonal effects (estrogenic or progestogenic) from other sources are not reflected in test results. Therefore, health care professionals who specialize in the area of hormone balance often diagnose and correct estrogen dominance based on symptoms only.

Q How can an imbalance of estrogen and progesterone levels be restored to a proper ratio?

Balance can often be restored by eliminating the source of estrogen (if known) and/or by raising the body's progesterone levels with USP grade natural progesterone. Progesterone is a single, specific hormone made by the ovaries in women and by the testes in males. It is also produced in smaller amounts by the adrenals in both sexes. Progesterone is the precursor (building block) to many of the other hormones found in the body and is therefore responsible for a number of essential bodily functions. It is in a class by itself, not to be confused with its synthetic counterpart, progestins. Interestingly, the progesterone hormone can be duplicated in molecular structure and action when derived from plants such as soy and a specific type of wild yam through a series of processes known as hydrolyzation. The end-product, USP grade *natural* progesterone, can be extremely beneficial when used transdermally for preventing and/or treating symptoms and conditions resulting from estrogen dominance due to its molecular structure being identical to the progesterone which the body itself manufactures.

Q Why not just use a progestin like Provera?

Progestins are all together different from the progesterone made within our bodies and the USP grade plant derived natural progesterone found in progesterone cream. While progestins are made from actual progesterone, their molecular structure is altered in order for them to become patentable by drug companies. As a result, progestins do not "physically" resemble progesterone, nor do they "act" like progesterone either. In fact, because of the significant difference in the molecular structure of progestins as compared to endogenous progesterone and natural progesterone, a fact our bodies are quick to recognize and respond to, progestins are associated with a long list of side effects and risk factors, some of which are potentially serious. These include but are not limited to menstrual irregularities, breast changes, insomnia, headaches, depression, fluid retention, cardiovascular events, strokes, and cancer.

Q Wouldn't it be more convenient just to use an oral form of natural progesterone instead of a cream?

God designed our bodies so that when our ovaries produce progesterone, they never deliver the hormone to the stomach. Yet, if we take a pill of any kind, it eventually ends up there. In the case of progesterone, which is fat-soluble, when taken orally it is absorbed from the stomach or intestines and then delivered by the portal vein directly to the liver where it is broken down and released in bile. Therefore, about 80 to 90 percent of oral progesterone is lost in the bile or converted into unrecognizable substances that are not capable of being utilized as actual progesterone.

Being fat-soluble, natural progesterone is best absorbed and more efficiently utilized when administered transdermally. Upon absorption through the fat layer below the skin, it directly enters the bloodstream, allowing for optimal bioavailability and systemic distribution throughout the entire body.

Q Not everything that is "natural" is considered "safe." How can I feel safe using natural progesterone?

For one thing, with all that we know regarding the dangers linked to synthetic estrogen and progestin use, it is interesting that there are those who approach using natural progesterone with skepticism. It certainly doesn't get much worse when it comes to potential side effects and risk factors than with synthetic estrogen and progestin usage. So, what about *natural* progesterone?

In all of the research I have done on this subject, I have found no evidence of documented risks associated with the use of USP grade natural progesterone cream when taken as needed in recommended therapeutic doses. Because natural progesterone has the identical molecular structure as the progesterone made by the ovaries (endogenous progesterone), natural progesterone is recognized and utilized as the actual progesterone hormone within the body, unlike progestins. Due to progesterone being the precursor ("building block") to the other sex hormones as well as the adrenal corticosteroid hormones, it plays a significant role in a variety of important bodily functions. Unlike with progestins, natural progesterone *is* capable of acting as a precursor to these other hormones because it has the identical molecular make-up as endogenous progesterone. Finally, we know that when a woman is pregnant, she produces about ten to fifteen times the amount of progesterone she normally does. So, if progesterone were harmful, every pregnant woman would be affected. While you would surely want to avoid taking more than the recommended therapeutic dose of natural progesterone to avoid an imbalance of another kind, it is unlikely that doing so would pose a serious risk.

Q Have quality studies been performed demonstrating the safety and effectiveness of natural progesterone cream?

Yes – published in reputable medical journals and cited throughout the text of this book.

Q But in using natural progesterone, isn't estrogen being overlooked – especially for women in menopause and/or who no longer have ovaries? Isn't supplemental estrogen beneficial for preventing dementia, osteoporosis, and heart disease in postmenopausal women?

While a small percentage of women may require supplemental estrogen, studies indicate that most women make sufficient estrogen after menopause through the age of 80. In addition to the ovaries, our body also makes estrogen in the adrenal glands and estrogen may be stored for years in the fat tissue. Furthermore, women are often exposed to exogenous sources of estrogen from estrogenic substances (xenoestrogens) which can increase estrogen levels. However, for women who truly demonstrate a deficiency of estrogen, it may be beneficial to supplement with estrogen in a low dose, using one of the least carcinogenic forms of estrogen, and always in combination with *natural* progesterone - not progestins (as opposed to using estrogen alone or "unopposed"). For more information, see Chapter 27, "The Estrogen Question."

In regards to recommending estrogen or HRT for the prevention of dementia, osteoporosis, and heart disease - the latest research does not support doing so. On the contrary, it points out the potential health risks involved. For a comprehensive update on each of these issues, I encourage you to read the specific chapters providing sound rationales using the most current, reputable research available. Chapters include, "Menopause 101," "The Heart of the Matter: The Truth About HRT and Heart Disease," "No Bones About It: The TRUTH About Osteoporosis," and "Frightening Facts."

Q How do doctors feel about natural progesterone therapy and conventional hormone replacement therapy today?

The following are examples of some doctors' thoughts on natural progesterone and/or conventional hormone therapy:

- **Dr. Robert Gottesman, M.D.**, private practice physician, author of "A Progesterone Saga"

  See Chapter 2 – "A Physician's Perspective" for a complete version of his paper, "A Progesterone Saga."

- **Dr. Helene Leonetti, M.D.**, private practice physician and associate professor of obstetrics and gynecology at Temple University "I'd estimate that I've put over 12,000 patients on progesterone, and they almost universally adore it."

"The most striking positive changes I see when women use natural progesterone cream are fewer mood swings, fewer hot flashes, and better sleep."

"I always know which of my patients are using progesterone when I do a breast exam, because their breasts are soft as babies' 'tushes.' Only about one in 2000 women have fibrocysts that don't melt with progesterone..."

- **Dr. Jerome Check, M.D.**, professor of obstetrics and gynecology and division head of reproductive endocrinology and infertility at the University of Medicine and Dentistry of New Jersey/Robert Wood Johnson Medical School at Camden and medical and laboratory director for the Cooper Center of In Vitro Fertilization.

"Too often physicians will treat the infertility problem with strong medication or even surgery without checking progesterone levels first...But for many women, progesterone therapy has been effective in helping them to become pregnant and to carry the child to term. Only after this treatment is tried should more drastic procedures be considered."

- **Dr. J. Ron Eaker, M.D.**, OB/GYN, author of "Holy Hormones!"

"The use of natural progesterone is another popular approach to treating PMS...I have used the natural progesterone cream with success..."

"There is evidence that natural progesterone cream is helpful for many menopausal symptoms...Data supporting this is beginning to appear. Two papers at the recent meeting of the World Congress on Fertility and Sterility showed significant improvement in hot flashes for women using natural progesterone cream versus a placebo. There are many anecdotal reports of its effectiveness, and I suspect that more investigations will be forthcoming."

"I have used it [natural progesterone cream] in my practice, specifically for hot flashes and have seen reasonable improvement."

- **Dr. Stephen Cummings, M.D.**, private practice physician, author, researcher

"Why take it [HRT]? If it's for hot flashes, it's clear it works. If it's for the prevention of anything [else], it's not clear yet."

"Until the effectiveness of estrogen is clarified, treatments other than estrogen should be the first choice for older women with osteoporosis."

"Since women in their fifties who do not have osteoporosis have a relatively low risk of fracture, the benefit of long term treatment with estrogen to prevent bone loss and fractures may not exceed the risks."

- **Dr. Peter Eckhart, M.D.**, private practice physician from Woodland Park, Colorado

Dr.Eckhart uses natural progesterone therapy for patients with prostate cancer. Is involved in research using natural progesterone for the prostate.

- **Dr. Jesse Hanley, M.D.**, medical director of Malibu Health and Rehabilitation Center

She uses natural progesterone cream as the basis for treatment with patients experiencing PMS and menopause symptoms. She also believes that estrogen dominance is associated with prostate cancer.

- **Dr. David Zava, PhD**, highly respected breast cancer researcher for 30 years. Experienced in conducting and evaluating saliva hormone assays for obtaining accurate hormone level readings.

"Unopposed estrogen therapy is truly iatrogenic illness at its worst. In most cases the entire domino effect, from estrogen dominance to overgrowth of the endometrial lining, to hysterectomy, to severe hormone imbalance and estrogen dominance caused by supplementation with unopposed estrogens, to excessive and unnecessary medications for depression and anxiety, to bone loss, could have been avoided if these women had known to use progesterone from the beginning."

- **Dr. Dean Raffelock**, doctor of chiropractic care, diplomat in acupuncture and applied kinesiology, and a certified clinical nutritionist.

Dr. Raffelock routinely assesses patients for estrogen dominance symptoms and recommends progesterone for normalizing thyroid function. He has found that balancing hormones often normalizes thyroid function and resolves other estrogen dominance symptoms. Furthermore, Dr. Raffelock points out, "The use of estrogen compounds like Premarin and some forms of birth control pills can raise T4 levels and mask or hide a low thyroid problem."

- **Dr. Dan Thibodeau**, doctor of chiropractic – Beck-Thibodeau Chiropractic, Appleton, WI

"As a chiropractor, I have been recommending alternatives to estrogen therapy for the past thirteen years. In our office we treat hundreds of patients with hormonal imbalances. Many of these patients have benefited from herbs and natural progesterone. We routinely use muscle testing and Contact Reflex Analysis (CRA) to test the different organs of the body to determine if there are imbalances. We can then quickly evaluate if natural progesterone will improve the patient's situation."

- **Dr. Judy Ellefson**, doctor of chiropractic – Family & Sports Chiropractic, Appleton, WI

"Having dealt with hormone imbalance on a personal level for much of my life, it is a joy to have information available and products to recommend to my patients who want an alternative to HRT."

- **Dr. Roy Ostenson**, doctor of chiropractic – Appleton Chiropractic Clinic, Appleton, WI

  "Since utilizing Dr. John Lee's progesterone program, I have seen incredible positive life changes in many of my patients. Every female patient that comes into my office gets a copy of Dr. Lee's audiotape."

- **Dr. John Lee, M.D.**, physician, author and leading authority on natural hormone treatments. A graduate of University of Minnesota and Harvard Medical School.

  "I have seen the consistent benefits and safety of natural progesterone therapy... The full history of progesterone is yet to occur. The scientific progress in the discovery and understanding of this remarkable hormone within just this century is amazing, of course, but even more is yet to come. The era of natural progesterone is not over; it is merely emerging from the flood of progestins..."

APPENDIX B

Choosing Wisely: Selecting a Natural Progesterone Product

Without a doubt, as with vitamins and other natural supplements, there are hundreds of brands of natural progesterone cream to choose from. Thus, there can be a great deal of confusion regarding the purity of various manufacturers' creams. The following tips will offer a bit of help in choosing a quality product:

- **Research the product manufacturer.** *Bioavailability* of the progesterone molecule in particular is what greatly influences the absorption and efficacy of a natural progesterone cream. Many companies or aspiring entrepreneurs are hearing about the benefits of natural progesterone cream and are interested solely in a "get-rich-quick" opportunity. Use only a cream containing pure, U.S. Pharmacopoeia (USP) grade natural progesterone. Some products, advertised as "wild yam cream" or "natural progesterone," actually contain the precursor of progesterone (diosgenin) and not the actual progesterone molecule. The human body is unable to convert these precursor substances to progesterone. In other words, diosgenin needs to be converted to progesterone by a series of hydrolyzing processes before it is capable of being utilized to achieve the results mentioned in this book. When properly processed, the end product is of the same molecular configuration as the progesterone made by the human body. Our bodies then recognize it as a compatible substance, utilizing it in the same capacity as endogenous progesterone (progesterone manufactured by the body), resulting in the beneficial outcomes commonly experienced by those who use it.

- **Read labels!** As with most skin care and cosmetic products, some brands of progesterone cream are formulated with animal products and by-products (ex. lanolin) or petroleum derivatives (petrolatum, mineral oil, etc.). The molecules contained within these ingredients are too large to adequately penetrate skin pores and may also be considered a toxic estrogenic compound (see Chapter Four). Therefore, these products essentially coat the skin with a "film," sealing it off. This results in inefficient or even impossible absorption of the natural progesterone and other beneficial ingredients, while also leaving behind toxic by-products. In other words, even if a product is formulated with therapeutic substances like natural progesterone, Aloe Vera, or Vitamin E, when it also contains a *petroleum derivative*, the skin is unable to absorb the beneficial ingredients properly, and you will therefore miss out on their inherent benefits. By becoming a "label reader," you will be surprised to learn how many skin care and cosmetics (even those considered "high-end") contain animal and/or petroleum derivatives as they are commonly used as "cheap fillers" in these products.

- **Know your "numbers."** Make sure the progesterone cream you use contains the recommended 1.6 percent cream with 450-500 mg of progesterone per ounce, giving you 15-20 mg of natural progesterone per 1/4 teaspoon dose. Supplementing with a cream that contains a higher or lower than recommended dose may not contribute to hormone balance.

- **Look for a metered-dose pump container.** Creams available in a metered dose pump container are optimal for several reasons. For one thing, this type of container ensures that the potent components of the cream remain active until gone. Research clearly indicates that exposure to light (due to repetitive opening of a "jar-style" container) and bacteria (present on fingers and hands when "dipping" into a container) can deactivate the fragile organic compounds that make natural progesterone cream effective. In fact, those who use natural progesterone cream from a jar often notice their symptoms reappear as they near the end of the container as a result of the deactivation of active ingredients. With a pump-style dispenser this phenomenon is avoided, assuring that your natural progesterone will be "good to the last drop!"

Furthermore, metered dose pump packaging lends to ease and accuracy in delivering the recommended 1/4 teaspoon (15-20mg) dose per application. There is no measuring or "guessing" involved as there is with "jars" or "tubes" of natural progesterone.

For a current listing of quality sources of natural progesterone, please consult Dr. John Lee, M.D.'s website – johnleemd.com. There are many quality sources of natural progesterone cream.

Whatever progesterone product you decide upon, it is important to recognize that God designed each of us uniquely. As with any medication or therapy, responses will vary. Natural progesterone therapy may not be "the answer" for everyone. Factors leading to the development of symptoms or conditions vary from person to person. Depending on a variety of factors, namely the existence and extent of estrogen dominance, natural progesterone will vary as to how and when it "works." While some individuals are able to detect a change in symptoms or in how they feel within the first month, others may go several months before noticing a difference. In the same way, while some individuals experience drastic responses, others report only mild changes. Finally, as with any therapy or lifestyle change, it is wise to inform your health care practitioner of your educated decision to supplement with natural progesterone.

APPENDIX C

Recommended Reading

For more on the subject of hormone balance please refer to:

- "What Your Doctor May Not Tell You About Menopause" by Dr. John Lee, M.D.

- "What Your Doctor May Not Tell You About Pre-menopause" by Dr. John Lee, M.D.

- "What Your Doctor May Not Tell You About Breast Cancer" by Dr. John Lee, M.D. and Dr. David Zava, PhD

- "The Estrogen Alternative" by Raquel Martin

To the Reader

The content of this book is meant to provide you with information that may be useful in attaining optimal health. Nothing is intended for use as instruction, a prescription, or as medical advice. No action or inaction should be taken solely on the content I have provided but rather one should consult with a trusted health care professional. It is always wise to inform your health care provider of your desire to implement any changes in your lifestyle, especially if you have an existing health condition or are taking medications of any kind. The information and opinions provided are believed to be accurate and sound based on my best judgment and research available. Keep in mind that health decisions are best resolved with a partnership between a well-informed patient and trusted health care provider.

REFERENCE LIST

Chapter One – Dear Doctor...

1. ***Merriam-Webster's Ninth Collegiate Dictionary.*** (1983). Springfield, MA: Merriam Webster.

2. ***Centers for Disease Control and Prevention.*** (1997). National ambulatory medical care survey (NAMCS). National Center for Health Statistics. Hyattville, MD.

3. ***Health Care Financing Administration.*** (1997). Statistical report on medical care. (HCFA-2082). Baltimore, MD.

4. ***Shuster, M. H.*** (2001). There is more than one way: the blending of traditional medicine with alternative care is growing significantly. Foxlife, 5 (4), 14.

5. ***Thedacare introduces holistic health initiative.*** (2001, March). At Heart, 6 (12), 9.

6. ***Integrated medicine for your health.*** (2002, Winter Edition). Healthy Balance, 7.

7. ***LaRoi, H.*** (2001, September 30). Women need to rethink priorities. The Post-Crescent, p. D-8.

8. *Lee, John R.* (1996). What your doctor may not tell you about menopause (p. xxiii). New York: Warner Books.

Chapter Two – A Physician's Perspective

1. *Gottesman, Robert* (1999). A progesterone saga.

Chapter Three – Progesterone, Progestins, & Natural Progesterone: Clearing Up the Confusion

1. *Lee, John R.* (1993). Natural progesterone: the multiple roles of a remarkable hormone (p. 38). Sebastopol, CA: BLL Publishing.

2. *Ibid.,* 5

3. *Ibid.,* 3-11.

4. *Gottesman, Robert* (2000). A progesterone saga.

5. *Lee, John R.* (1993). Natural progesterone: the multiple roles of a remarkable hormone (p.20). Sebastopol, CA: BLL Publishing.

6. *National Toxicology Program (NTP).* (1988). Fourth Annual Report on Carcinogens.

7. **Shairer, C., Lubin, J., Trois, R., Sturgeon, S., Brinton, L., Hoover, R.** (2001). Menopausal estrogen and estrogen-progestin replacement therapy and breast cancer risk. Journal of the American Medical Association, 283 (4), 485-491. Lee, John R. (1993). Natural progesterone: the multiple roles of a remarkable hormone (p.76). Sebastopol, CA: BLL Publishing.

8. **Lee, John R.** (1993). Natural progesterone: the multiple roles of a remarkable hormone (p. 76). Sebastopol, CA: BLL Publishing.

9. **Eaker, R.** (1999). Holy hormones! (p. 178). Enumclaw, WA: Winepress Publishing.

10. **Leonetti, H. B., Longo, S., Anasti, J.,** (1999). Transdermal progesterone cream for vasomotor symptoms and postmenopausal bone loss. Obstetrics & Gynecology, 94 (2), 225-228.

11. **Anasti, J., Leonetti, H.B., Wilson, K.J.,** (2001). Topical progesterone cream has an antiproliferative effect on estrogen-stimulated endometrium. Obstetrics & Gynecology, 97 (4 Suppl 1), 10s.

12. **Ibid.**

13. ***Progesterone cream protects the uterus from the effects of estrogen.*** (2001, June). John R. Lee, M.D. Medical Letter, 6.

Chapter Four – An Introduction to Estrogen Dominance: The Concept and Causes

1. ***Lee, John R.*** (1999). What your doctor may not tell you about premenopause (p. 324). NY: Warner Books.

2. ***Ibid.***

3. ***Ibid., 216***

4. ***Vastag, B.*** (2001). CDC unveils first report on toxins in people. Journal of the American Medical Association, 285 (14), 1827-1828.

5. ***Lee, John R.*** (1996). What your doctor may not tell you about menopause (p. 46). NY: Warner Books.

6. ***Lee, John R.*** (1999). What your doctor may not tell you about premenopause (p. 25). NY: Warner Books.

7. ***Ibid., 216-217.***

Chapter Five – Solving the PMS Puzzle

1. *Lee, John R.* (1999). What your doctor may not tell you about premenopause (p.136). NY: Warner Books.

2. *Lee, John R.* (1996). What your doctor may not tell you about menopause (p.98). NY: Warner Books.

3. *Slater, L.* (2001). Beyond prozac: new treatments, new hope. Rosie, 129 (10), 130.

4. *Eaker, R.J.* (1999). Holy hormones! (p. 97). Enumclaw, WA: Winepress Publishing.

Chapter Six – "Not Tonight, Honey – I Have a Headache"

1. *Mitchell, T.* (2000, October 6-8). Fighting headaches is a pain. USA Weekend, 4.

2. *Lee, John R.* (1996). What your doctor may not tell you about menopause (pp. 251-252). NY: Warner Books.

3. *Lee, John R.* (1999). What your doctor may not tell you about premenopause (p. 177). NY: Warner Books.

Chapter Seven – The "Low-Down" on Unexplained Weight Gain & other Symptoms of Low Thyroid

1. *Lee, John R.* (1993). Natural progesterone: the multiple roles of a remarkable hormone (pp. 51, 81). Sebastopol, CA: BLL Publishing.

2. *Arafah, B.M.* (2000). Increased need for thyroxine in women with hypothyroidism during estrogen therapy. New England Journal of Medicine, 344 (23), 1743-1749.

3. *Lee, John R.* (1999). What your doctor may not tell you about premenopause (pp. 187-188). NY: Warner Books.

4. *Lee, John R.* (1996). What your doctor may not tell you about menopause (pp. 38-41, 204-207). NY: Warner Books.

5. *Lee, John R.* (1999). What your doctor may not tell you about premenopause (pp. 47, 60). NY: Warner Books.

6. *Arafah, B.M.* (2001). Increased need for thyroxine in women with hypothyroidism during estrogen therapy. New England Journal of Medicine, 344 (23), 1743-1749.

7. *Patterns of hormonal imbalance, cortisol effects, and more.* (2001, February). John R. Lee, M.D. Medical Letter, 6.

8. *Lee, John R.* (1996). What your doctor may not tell you about menopause (pp. 146-148). NY: Warner Books.

9. *Reading blood tests for optimal ranges.* (2001, March). John R. Lee, M.D. Medical Letter, 6.

Chapter Eight – Fibromyalgia Facts

1. *Trivison, S., Gerstung, J.* (2000). Get smart! Get help…from the experts (Cassette Recording, Tape 3). Scottsdale, AZ: Smart Radio.

2. *Ibid.*

Chapter Nine – Estrogen: A Chronic Fatigue Factor

1. *Lee, John R.* (1999). What your doctor may not tell you about premenopause (p. 50). NY: Warner Books.

2. *Ibid., 189-190.*

Chapter Ten – Fibrocystic Breast Facts

1. *Rice, C. W.* (2001, June). A natural solution for fibrocystic breast disease. Natural Muscle, 24.

2. *Rutter, C. M., Mandelson, M. T., Laya, M. B., Toplin, S.* (2001). Changes in breast density associated with initiation, discontinuation, and continuing use of hormone replacement therapy. Journal of the American Medical Association, 285 (2), 171-176.

3. *Progesterone cream protects the uterus from the effects of estrogen.* (2001, June). John R. Lee, M.D. Medical Letter, 6.

Chapter Eleven – Miscarriage & Infertility Insights

1. *Lee, John R.* (1996). What your doctor may not tell you about menopause (p. 106). NY: Warner Books.

2. *Ibid., 244.*

3. *Ibid., 245.*

4. *Graham, L.C.* (1989, February). Do you have a hormone shortage? Redbook, 16.

5. *Eisenstein, M.* (2000). Safer medicine. USA: CMI Press.

Chapter Twelve – Progesterone & the Postpartum Depression Connection

1. *O'Hara, M.W., Alloy, L.B.* (1994). Postpartum depression. NY: Springer-Verlag.

2. *Harris, B.* (1994). Maternity blues and major endocrine changes: Cadiff puerperal mood and hormone study II, Wales. British Medical Journal, 308, 949-953.

3. *Dalton, K.* (1990). Guide to progesterone for postnatal depression [Brochure].

Chapter Thirteen – Views on Vaginal Dryness & Low Libido

1. *Lee, J.R.* (1996). What your doctor may not tell you about menopause (p. 109). NY: Warner Books.

Chapter Fourteen – Hysterectomy or Not to Be?

1. *Lee, John R.* (1996). What your doctor may not tell you about menopause (p. 245). NY: Warner Books.

2. *Lee, John R.* (1999). What your doctor may not tell you about premenopause (p. 332). NY: Warner Books.

3. *Anasti, J., Leonetti, H.B., Wilson, K. J.* (2001). Topical progesterone cream has an antiproliferative effect on estrogen-stimulated endometrium. Obstetrics & Gynecology, 97 (4 Suppl 1), 10s.

4. *Lee, John R.* (1996). What your doctor may not tell you about menopause (p. 240). NY: Warner Books.

5. *Lee, John R.* (1993). Natural progesterone: the multiple roles of a remarkable hormone (p. 87). Sebastopol, CA: BLL Publishing.

6. *Wood, A.J.J.* (2001). Treatment of endometriosis. New England Journal of Medicine, 345 (4). 266-273.

7. *Lee, John R.* (1996). What your doctor may not tell you about menopause (p. 241). NY: Warner Books.

8. ***Lee, John R.*** (1999). What your doctor may not tell you about premenopause (pp. 192-193). NY: Warner Books.

9. ***Ibid., 194.***

10. ***And there's more*** (2001, May). The John R. Lee, M.D. Medical Letter, 8.

11. ***Anasti, J., Leonetti, H.B., Wilson, K.J.*** (2001). Topical progesterone cream has an antiproliferative effect on estrogen-stimulated endometrium. Obstetrics & Gynecology, 97 (4 Suppl 1), 10s.

12. ***Lee, John R.*** (1996). What your doctor may not tell you about menopause (p. 246). NY: Warner Books.

Chapter Fifteen – Gallbladder Grief

1. ***What your doctor may not tell you about gallbladder disease and bile flow.*** (2001, February). The John R. Lee, M.D. Medical Letter, 2-3.

2. ***Ibid.***

3. ***Ibid.***

4. ***Ibid.***

Chapter Sixteen – Estrogen Dominance & Autoimmune Disorders: A Likely Link

1. *Lee, John R.* (1996). What your doctor may not tell you about menopause (p. 148). NY: Warner Books.

2. *Lee, John R.* (1999). What your doctor may not tell you about premenopause (pp. 180-181). NY: Warner Books.

Chapter Seventeen – The "Skinny" on Skin Conditions

1. *Schiff, G., Wisniewski, M., Bult, J., Parada, J., Aggarwal, H., Schwartz, D.* (2001). Improving inpatient antibiotic prescribing: insights from participation in a national collaborative. The Joint Commission Journal on Quality Improvement, 27 (8), 387-399.

2. *Twersky, O.* (2000). Controversial acne drug could get popped: Congress to investigate reports linking accutane with depression, suicide [Online], File: WebMD.lycos.com/content/article/1685.51057.

3. *Lee, John R.* (1996). What your doctor may not tell you about menopause (p. 252). NY: Warner Books.

4. *Ibid., 253.*

5. *Ibid.*

Chapter Eighteen – Precocious Pubescence

1. *Herman-Giddens, M.E., Slora, E.J., Wasserman, R.C., Bourdony, C. J., Bhapkar, M.V., Koch, G.G., Hasemeier, C.M.* (1997). Secondary sexual characteristics and menses in young girls seen in office practice: A study from the Pediatric Research in Office Settings Network. Pediatrics, 99, (4), 505-512.

2. *Lee, John R.* (1996). What your doctor may not tell you about menopause (pp. 59-60). NY: Warner Books.

Chapter Nineteen – Frightening Facts

1. *Simone, C., Simone, N., Simone II, C., Pallante, M.* (2000). The role of glucarate in cancer treatment. International Journal of Integrative Medicine, 2 (5), 42-48.

2. ***Reinhardt Reiss, J. and Ravinett Martin, A.*** (2000) Breast cancer 2000: An update on facts, figures, and issues. (p. 3). The Breast Cancer Fund.

3. ***Simone, C., Simone, N., Simone II, C., Pallante, M.*** (2000). The role of glucarate in cancer treatment. International Journal of Integrative Medicine, 2 (5), 42-48.

4. ***Ibid., 42.***

5. ***Groopman, J.*** (2001, June 4). The thirty-year war: Have we been fighting cancer the wrong way? The New Yorker, 52-63.

6. ***Ibid.***

7. ***Bailar, J.C., Smith, E.M.*** (1986). Progress against cancer? New England Journal of Medicine, 314 (19), 1226-1232.

8. ***Chang, K.J., Lee, T.T.Y., Linares-Cruz, G., Fournier, S., de Lignieres, B.*** (1995). Influences of percutaneous administration of estradiol and progesterone on human breast epithelial cell cycle in vivo. Fertility and Sterility, 63, 785-791.

9. ***Anasti, J., Leonetti, H.B., Wilson, K.J.*** (2001). Topical progesterone cream has an anti-proliferative effect of estrogen-stimulated endometrium. Obstetrics & Gynecology, 97 (4 Suppl 1), 10s.

10. ***Report on carcinogens*** (2000, December 15), National Toxicology Program (NTP).

Chapter Twenty – Keeping Abreast of Breast Cancer

1. ***Greenlee, R.T., Murray, T., Bolden, S., Wingo, P.A.*** (2000). Cancer statistics 2000. Cancer – A Cancer Journal for Clinicians, 50 (1), 7-33.

2. ***Reinhardt Reiss, J. and Ravinett Martin, A.*** (2000). Breast cancer 2000: An update on facts, figures, and issues. (p. 4). The Breast Cancer Fund.

3. ***Simone, C., Simone, N., Simone II, C., Pallante, M.*** (2000). The role of glucarate in cancer treatment. International Journal of Integrative Medicine, 2 (5), 42-48.

4. ***Cowan, L.D., Gordis, L., Tonascia, J.A., Jones, G.S.*** (1981). Breast cancer incidence

in women with a history of progesterone (endogenous) deficiency. American Journal of Epidemiology, 114 (2), 209-217.

5. *Chang, K.J., Lee, T.T.Y., Linares-Cruz, G., Fournier, S., de Lignieres, B.* (1995). Influences of percutaneous administration of estroadiol on human breast epithelial cell cycle in vivo. Fertility and Sterility, 63 (4), 785-791.

6. *Lee, John, R.* (1999). What your doctor may not tell you about premenopause (p. 212). NY: Warner Books.

7. *Ibid., 213.*

8. *Breast hormone receptors and breast cancer.* (2001, January). The John R. Lee, M.D. Medical Letter, 2.

9. *Ibid.*

10. *Colburn, T., Dumanoski, D., Myers, J.P.* (1997). Our stolen future. NY: Penguin Books.

11. *Wolff, M.S., Collman, G.W., Barrett, J.C., Huff, J.* (1996). Breast cancer and environmental risk factors: epidemiological

and experimental findings. Annual Review of Pharmacology and Toxicology, 36, 573-596.

12. *Clemons, M., Goss, P.* (2001). Estrogen and the risk of breast cancer. New England Journal of Medicine, 344 (4), 276-285.

13. *Davis, D.L., Axelrod, D., Gaynor, M., Bailey, L.* (1997). Environmental influences on breast cancer risk. Science and Medicine, 4 (3), 56-63.

14. *Lee, John, R.* (1999). What your doctor may not tell you about premenopause (p. 223). NY: Warner Books.

15. *Ibid., 223-224.*

16. *Ibid.*

17. *Clemons, M., Goss, P.* (2001). Estrogen and the risk of breast cancer. New England Journal of Medicine, 344 (4), 276-285.

18. *Bergkvist, L., H-O. Adami, I., Persson, R., Hoover, R., Shairer, C.* (1989). The risk of breast cancer after estrogen and estrogen-progestin replacement. New England Journal of Medicine, 321 (5), 293-299.

19. *Shairer, C., Lubin, J., Trossi, R., Sturgeon, S., Brinton, L., Hoover, R.* (2000). Menopausal estrogen and estrogen-progestin replacement therapy and breast cancer risk. Journal of the American Medical Association, 283 (4), 485-491.

20. *Grabick, D.M., Hartman, L.C., Cerhan, J.R., Vierkant, R.A., Therneau, T.M., Vachon, C.M., Olson, J.E., Couch, F.J., Anderson, K.E., Pankratz, S., Sellers, T.A.* (2000). Risk of breast cancer with oral contraceptive use in women with a family history of breast cancer. Journal of the American Medical Association, 284 (14), 1791-1798.

Chapter Twenty-One – Ovarian Cancer Makes the Headlines

1. *Rodriguez, C., Patel, A.V., Calle, E.E., Jacob, E.J., Thun, M.J.* (2001). Estrogen replacement therapy and ovarian cancer mortality in a large prospective study of US women. Journal of the American Medical Association, 285 (11), 1460-1465.

2. *Rodriguez, C., Calle, E.E., Coates, R.J., Miracle-McMahill, H.L., Thun, M.J., Heath, C.W.* (1995). American Journal of Epidemiology, 141 (9), 828-835.

3. *Lee, John R.* (1999). What your doctor may not tell you about premenopause (pp. 239-240). NY: Warner Books.

4. *Cancer facts and figures.* (1999). American Cancer Society.

5. *Rodriguez, C., Calle,E.E., Jacobs, E., Patel, A., Thun, M.* (2001). Relationship between postmenopausal hormone replacement therapy and ovarian cancer (Reply to letter to the editor). Journal of the American Medical Association, 285 (24), 3090.

Chapter Twenty-Two – The Problematic Prostate

1. Greenlee, R.T., Murray, T., Bolden, S., Wingo, P.A. (2000). Cancer statistics 2000. Cancer – A Cancer Journal for Clinicians, 50 (1), 7-33.

2. Eckhart, P. (1997). Prostate hormone therapy: An invitation for a clinical trial for prostate cancer treatment [Online]. File: dreckhart.hypermart.net. Woodland Park, CO: Prostate Hormone Therapy.

Chapter Twenty-Three – "Menopause 101"

1. ***Low Dog, T., Riley, D., Carter, T.*** (2001). An integrative approach to menopause. Alternative Therapies, 7 (4), 45-55.

2. ***Lee, John R.*** (1996). What your doctor may not tell you about menopause (p. 70). NY: Warner Books.

3. ***Ibid.***

4. ***Ibid.***

5. **Lee, John R.** (1999) What your doctor may not tell you about premenopause (p.51) . NY: Warner Books.

6. **Martin, R.** (1998). The estrogen alternative (p. 129). Rochester, VT: healing Arts Press.

7. **Lee, John R.** (1996). What your doctor may not tell you about menopause (p 123). NY: Warner Books.

8. ***Ibid.,*** 246.

9. ***Ibid.,*** 22-23

10. ***Ibid.***

11. **Rubin, R.** (2001, June 13). Hormone therapy: Doubts grow. USA Today, p. 2A.

12. **Rexrode, K., Manson, J.** (2001). Postmenopausal hormone replacement therapy: No cause for celebration. Journal of the American Medical Association, 287 (5), 461-462.

13. **Rubin, R.** (2001, June 13). Hormone therapy: Doubts grow. USA Today, p. 2A.

14. **Grady, D., Cummings, S.** (2001). Postmenopausal hormone therapy for prevention of fractures: How good is the evidence? Journal of the American Medical Association, 285 (22), 2909-2910.

15. **Revised cholesterol guidelines.** (2001, July). Harvard Heart Letter, 11 (11), 6-7.

16. **Leblanc, E.S., Nelson, H.** (2001). Hormone replacement therapy and cognition in postmenopausal women. Journal of the American Medical Association, 285 (23), 2975-2975.

17. **Eaker, J. R.** (1999). Holy hormones! (p. 178) Enumclaw, WA: Winepress Publishing.

18. *Leonetti, H., Longo, S., Anasti, J.* (1999). Transdermal progesterone cream for vasomotor symptoms and postmenopausal bone loss. Obstetrics & Gynecology, 94 (2), 225-228.

19. *Anasti, J., Leonetti, H., Wilson, K.J.* (2001). Topical progesterone cream has anti-proliferative effect on estrogen-stimulated endometrium. Obstetrics & Gyneology, 97 (4 Suppl 1), 10s.

20. *Ibid.*

21. *Eaker, J.R.,* (1999). Holy hormones! (p. 178). Enumclaw, WA: Winepress Publishing.

22. *Progesterone cream protects the uterus from the effects of estrogen.* (2001, June). John R. Lee, M.D. Medical Letter, 6.

Chapter Twenty-Four – The Heart of the Matter: The TRUTH about HRT and Heart Disease

1. *Mosca, L., Collins, P., Herrington, D., Mendelsohn, M., Pasternak, R., Robertson, R., Schenck-Gustafsson, K., Smith, S., Taubert, K., Wenger, N.* (2001). Hormone replacement therapy and cardiovascular disease: A statement for healthcare

professionals from the American Heart Association. Circulation, 104 (4), 499-502.

2. **Rubin, R.** (2001, June 13). Hormone therapy: Doubts grow. USA Today, 2A.
3. **Mitka, M.** (2001). New advice for women patients about hormone therapy and the heart. Journal of the American Medical Association, 286 (8), 907.

4. **A second look at HRT and heart attack prevention.** (1998, November). Harvard Health Letter, 24 (1), 7.

5. **Ibid.**

6. **More questions on estrogens.** (2000, June). Harvard Heart Letter, 10 (10), 6-7.

7. **Rubin, R.** (2001, June 13). Hormone therapy: Doubts grow. USA Today, 2A.

8. **Herrington, D., Reboussin, D., Brosnihan, B., Sharp, P., Shumaker, S., Snyder, T., Furberg, C., Kowalchuk, G., Stuckey, T., Rogers, W., Givens, D., Waters, D.** (2000). Effects of estrogen replacement on the progression of coronary artery atherosclerosis. New England Journal of Medicine, 343 (8), 522-529.

9. *Will statins unseat estrogens?* (2000, November). Harvard Heart Letter, 11 (3), 1-3.

10. *Manson, J.E., Martin, K.A.* (2001). Postmenopausal hormone replacement therapy. New England Journal of Medicine, 345 (1), 34-40.

11. *Prior, J.C. Letter. New England Journal of Medicine, 326, 705-706.*

12. *Rubin, R.* (2001, June 13). Hormone therapy: Doubts grow. USA Today, 2A.

13. *Lee, John R.* (1996). What your doctor may not tell you about menopause (p. 254). NY: Warner Books.

14. *Ibid., 197.*

15. *Verschuren, M., Jacobs, D., Bloemberg, B., Kromhout, D., Menotti, A., Aravanis, C., Blackburn, H., Buzina, R., Dontas, A., Fidanza, F., Karvonen, M., Nedeljkovic, S., Nissinen, A., Toshima, H.* (1995). Serum total cholesterol and long-term coronary heart disease mortality in different cultures. Journal of the American Medical Association, 274 (2), 131-136.

16. **Manson, J.E., Martin, K.A.** (2001). Postmenopausal hormone replacement therapy. New England Journal of Medicine, 345 (1), 34-40.

17. **Revised cholesterol guidelines.** (2001, July). Harvard Heart Letter, 11 (11), 6-7.

18. **Rubin, R.** (2001, June 13). Hormone therapy: Doubts grow. USA Today, 2A.

Chapter Twenty-Five – No Bones About It: The Truth About Estrogen and Osteoporosis

1. **Rubin, R.** (2001, June 13). Hormone therapy: Doubts grow. USA Today, 2A.

2. **Prior, J.C., Vigna, Y., Alojada, N.** (1990), Spinal bone loss and ovulatory disturbances. International Journal of Gynecology and Obstetrics, 34, 253-256.

3. **Grady, D., Cummings, S.** (2001). Postmenopausal hormone therapy for prevention of fractures: How good is the evidence? Journal of the American Medical Association, 285 (22), 2909-2910.

4. **Rubin, R.** (2001, June 13). Hormone therapy: Doubts grow. USA Today, 2A. Ibid.

5. *Grady, D., Cummings, S.* (2001). Postmenopausal hormone therapy for prevention of fractures: How good is the evidence? Journal of the American Medical Association, 285 (22), 2909-2910.

6. *Baran, D.* (2000). Osteoporosis: Which current treatment reduces fracture risk? Cleveland Clinic Journal of Medicine, 67 (10), 702-703.

7. *Nerhood, Robert,* (2001). Making a decision about ERT/HRT. Postgraduate Medicine, 109 (3), 167-178.

8. *Cauley, J.A., Black, D.M., Barrett-Connor, E., Harris, F., Shields, K., Applegate, W., Cummings, S*. (2001). Effects of hormone replacement therapy on clinical fractures and height loss: The heart and estrogen/progestin replacement study (HERS). American Journal of Medicine, 110 (6), 442-449.

9. *Rubin, R.* (2001, June 13). Hormone therapy: Doubts grow. USA Today, 2A.

10. *Lee, John R.* (1996). What your doctor may not tell you about menopause (p. 151). NY: Warner Books.

11. *Ibid., 173.*

12. *Letter.* (2001, March). John R. Lee M.D. Medical Letter, 7.

Chapter Twenty-Six – The Problem with "the Pill" and other Chemical Contraceptives

1. *Berger, G.S., Goldstein, M., Fuerst, M.* (1995). The couple's guide to fertility (Revised Edition). NY: Doubleday Press.
2. *Einstein, M.* (2000). Excerpt from safer medicine. [Online]. File: homefirst.com/pill.html. CMI Press.

3. *Physicians Desk Reference* (2000). Montvale, NJ: Medical Economics Company, Inc., pp. 2172-2198.

4. *Chemical birth control increases risks.* (2001, September/October). The John R. Lee, M.D. Medical Letter, 4.

5. *Lee, John R.* (1999). What your doctor may not tell you about premenopause (p. 203). NY: Warner Books.

6. *Clemons, M., Goss, P.* (2001). Estrogen and the risk of breast cancer. New England Journal of Medicine, 344 (4), 276-285.

7. *Grabick, D.M., Hartman, L.C., Cerhan, J.R., Vierkant, R.A., Thernau, T.M., Vachon, C.M., Olson, J.E., Couch, F.J., Anderson, K.E., Pankratz, S., Sellers, T.A.* (2000). Risk of breast cancer with oral contraceptive use with family history of breast cancer. Journal of the American Medical Association, 284 (14), 1791-1798.

8. *And there's more (2001, May). The John R. Lee, M.D. Medical Letter, 8.*

Chapter Twenty-Seven – The Estrogen Question

1. *The use of postmenopausal estrogen replacement.* (2001, January). The John R. Lee, M.D. Medical Letter, 2.

2. *Progesterone cream protects the uterus from the effects of estrogen.* (2001, June). The John R. Lee, M.D. Medical Letter, 5-6.

3. *Lee, John R.* (1996). What your doctor may not tell you about menopause (p. 209). NY: Warner Books.

4. *Low Dog, T., Riley, D., Carter, T.* (2001). An integrative approach to menopause. Alternative Therapies, 7 (4), 45-55.

5. ***Cutler, S.J., Cutler, J.A., Cutler, H.G.***
   (2000, September). Phytoestrogens in
   hormone replacement therapy. Pharmacist,
   56-64.

6. ***Lee, John R.*** (1996). What your doctor may
   not tell you about menopause (p.125). NY:
   Warner Books

7. ***Patterns of hormonal imbalances, cortisol
   effects, and more.*** (2001, February). The
   John R. Lee, M.D. Medical Letter, 5-6.

8. ***Lee, John R.*** (1999). What your doctor may
   not tell you about premenopause (p.51). NY:
   Warner Books.

Chapter Twenty-Eight – Why a Cream?

1. ***Lee, John R.*** (1996). What your doctor may
   not tell you about menopause (p. 324). NY:
   Warner Books.

2. ***Ibid.***

Chapter Twenty-Nine – The "Bigger Picture:" Other Factors of Optimal Health

1. ***Kahn, S.*** (2001, October). Beat the odds.
   Great Life, 32-35.

Index

Libido (see also Sex drive)
19, 60, 80, 85-86, 97,
105, 113-115, 118,
185, 197, 230, 267
Liver 246, 254, 271
Longo, Santo 52, 195
Lupus erythematosis (see
also Autoimmune
diseases) 136
Luteal phase failure 104
Lymphoma 167

Magnesium 76-77, 205,
218-220, 235
Mammogram 100
Manson, JoAnn 192
Masculinizing effects 50,
191
Mastectomy 171
Meat (see Diet)
Medroxyprogesterone
acetate (see Provera)
Men 57, 118, 131, 153, 178
Menopausal
symptoms (see also
Anxiety; Hot flashes;
Low libido; Sleep
disorders; Vaginal
dryness) 10, 20, 32,
37, 52, 54, 89, 105,
184, 186, 189, 194-
197, 213, 243-248,
277-279 women
50, 52, 62, 114, 119,
154, 174-176, 184,

195, 197, 200-202,
208, 211, 242, 274
Menopause (see also
Menopausal
symptoms;
Menopausal women)
60, 62, 100, 105, 124,
164, 173, 183-198,
203, 214, 223, 232,
246, 248, 274-275,
277-279
Menses (see also Menstrual
cycle; Menstruation;
period) early (see also
Precocious puberty)
143, 163
Menstrual
cramps 21, 61, 65, 69,
73, 120, 237-238
cycle 21, 74, 119,
122, 143-145, 161
irregularities 50, 267,
270
Menstruation (see also
Menses; Period;
Menstrual cycle) 62,
69, 104, 143-145
Migraines (see Headaches)
Mineral oil 49, 60, 252, 285
Miscarriage 103-107
Mitchell, Tedd 75
Mitochondria 96
Mood swings 54, 69-71, 73,
96, 105, 110, 185,
197, 239, 244, 276
Mosca, Lori 200

Vaginal dryness 113-115,
185, 197, 230, 239,
244, 247,
Vegetables (see Diet)
Visco, Fran 151
Vitamins (see also
Supplements) 120,
218-221, 235

Water 133, 257
Water retention (see also
Bloating; Edema;
Fluid retention) 69,
105, 248, 266,
Weight 64, 80-82, 87-88,
133, 210
Gain 19, 80-83, 85,
87-88, 97, 105, 225,
235, 248, 267
Weight-bearing exercise (see
Exercise)
West, Stanley 117
Wild yam 51, 269, 284
Wilson, K.J. 119
Wilson, Robert 188-189
Women's Health Initiative
(WHI) 203, 205, 218
World Health Organization
(WHO) 58, 63, 266

Xenoestrogens (see also
Environmental toxins;
Estrogenic
compounds) 60, 145,
274

Yeast infections (see also
Candida) 138. 234

Zava, David 86, 161, 247,
279
Zinc 47, 70-71, 96, 218